Living the Gi Diet

Rick Gallop

Delicious recipes and real life strategies to **lose weight and keep it off**

This edition first published in Great Britain in 2004 by:
Virgin Books
Thames Wharf Studios
Rainville Road
London W6 9HA

First published by Random House Canada

This edition published by arrangement with Random House Canada,
a division of Random House of Canada Limited

A catalogue record for the book is available from the British Library.

ISBN: 0 7535 0882 6

Designed by Smith & Gilmour

Printed and bound in Spain by Bookprint, S.L., Barcelona

Contents

For the thousands of readers who have shared their stories and successes with me and who gave me the inspiration and motivation to write this book.

Introduction

In 2002, I launched my first book, *The G.I. Diet,* with some trepidation. It wasn't the diet's effectiveness that I was worried about – far from it. I knew from personal experience that it was the best weight-loss programme available. The book was based on the latest scientific research and had been endorsed by a number of physicians. I myself had lost twenty pounds on it after all but giving up hope of ever slimming down. What did concern me was that it might get lost in the sea of diet books crowding bookshop shelves – books that were full of empty promises, that promoted diets that were dangerously unhealthy or that simply did not work.

I wanted to let people know the real cause of their weight problem and that they could lose the extra pounds easily, without having to perform difficult mathematical calculations or having to go hungry. I'm convinced that the reason we are gaining more weight than ever before is because they have simply been given the wrong information. The truth is you can eat as much or even more than you currently do and still slim down. All you have to do is choose the right foods.

Fortunately, people took notice of *The G.I. Diet* and it clearly hit a chord with them. The book became an international bestseller, and tens of thousands of readers have lost weight on the programme! It is so rewarding to receive everyone's e-mails describing their successes – and they are the real motivation behind my writing this second book, *Living the G.I. Diet*. I wanted to provide even more information and lots of wonderful recipes to help you continue losing pounds or to maintain your new weight.

Dear Rick,

I tried several diet plans throughout the last thirty years . . . .
None of them worked for any length of time. And all the weight
I lost came back threefold.

I was riding my exercise bike and watching the news when
the health segment came on. They talked about *The G.I. Diet* and
raved about the results some people had had with it. Best of all,
they talked about the fact that the diet would lower cholesterol,
and keep your sugar levels low. This sounded good to me, as my
family has a history of diabetes, and I was a very good candidate
to develop this disease in the next few years.

So I went out and purchased the book and began to read it
that night. I couldn't put it down! It all made perfect sense and
was written in a way that was easily understood, and best of all:
NO MEASURING ANY FOOD!

I have lost a total of 4½ stones, and have dropped from a
size 28 (which was a very tight 28) to a size 18! More important
than the weight loss is the fact that my last blood tests done
by my doctor were unbelievable. My cholesterol levels have
dropped dramatically and I am now in the normal levels – a big
change from almost having to go on medication to control it! I
feel that the G.I. Diet is the best! The world would not be in such
dire straits with the obesity problems if everyone went G.I.

Thanks for listening.

Pamela

For those of you who didn't read *The G.I. Diet*, I've started this book with a short outline of its principles. This summary will give you everything you need to get started on the programme right away. If you feel, however, that you need a more detailed explanation, you may want to read my first book. Those of you who are already familiar with the programme can read the summary for a quick refresher or just skip over it. I should mention, though, that the G.I. Diet Food Guide on page 20 has been expanded to include even more foods than appeared in the first book.

I've also decided to enlist the help of experts in writing this book. I've asked my wife, Dr Ruth Gallop, to write a chapter on how to deal with the emotional reasons why we eat. She is a professor and an international authority on childhood trauma and its impact on our behaviour as adults. Though not all of us have suffered trauma, most of us do use food for reasons other than physiological need. If you have a bad day at work, do you buy a box of chocolates on your way home? If you're alone on a Saturday night, do you indulge in a tub of Häagen-Dazs ice cream? Ruth will tell you how to ease yourself out of the habit of turning to food for comfort when you are feeling stressed or depressed.

I've also asked Emily Richards, the co-host of a popular North American TV cooking series, to create a cornucopia of delicious green- and yellow-light recipes for breakfast, lunch, snacks, dinner and yes, even dessert. You can eat a wide variety of flavourful, appealing dishes on this programme and never feel as though you are on a diet. In fact, many of them are sure to become family favourites.

To further motivate you, I've shared some of the e-mails I've received from people who are on the G.I. Diet. Their stories are often moving and truly inspiring. I am so proud of them and so grateful for their feedback. I hope that their experiences will help you as you embark on your journey to a new, slim you!

The G.i. Diet in a Nutshell

part
one

1 The Secret to Easy, Permanent Weight Loss

For years doctors, nutritionists and government officials have told us that the way to maintain a healthy weight is to eat a low-fat, high-carbohydrate diet. So if you've ever tried to lose weight, you've probably started by reducing the amount of fat that you eat. Instead of having bacon and eggs for breakfast, you switched to cornflakes with skimmed milk. Instead of eating a hamburger at lunch, you opted for chicken noodle soup and a slice of white bread without butter. Instead of snacking on potato chips, you munched on a couple of rice cakes. You made these healthier choices, felt good about yourself, and at the end of the month, you eagerly weighed yourself again – to find that you'd gained another two pounds! What happened?

Well, first of all, let's dispel a widely held myth: fat does not necessarily make you fat. Fat consumption in this country has remained virtually constant over the past ten years, while obesity numbers have rocketed. Obviously fat isn't the culprit. But that doesn't mean you can eat all the fatty foods you want. Most fats can be quite harmful to your health. It's alarming to read some of the popular diet books on the market today and find that they advocate eating lots of cream, cheese and steak. These foods are all high in saturated fat, which can thicken arteries, leading to heart attack and stroke. There is also increasing evidence that colon and prostate cancer as well as Alzheimer's are associated with high levels of saturated fats. These are definitely the 'bad' fats and are easily recognizable because they solidify at room temperature and almost always come from animal sources. There are two exceptions to this rule: coconut oil and palm oil are two vegetable oils that are also saturated. Because these oils are cheap, they are used in many snack foods, especially biscuits.

COOKING OILS/FATS

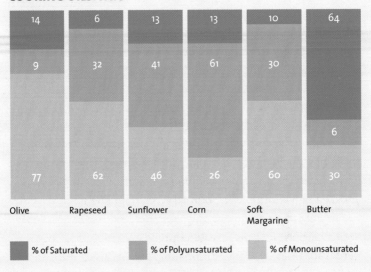

	Olive	Rapeseed	Sunflower	Corn	Soft Margarine	Butter
% of Saturated	14	6	13	13	10	64
% of Polyunsaturated	9	32	41	61	30	6
% of Monounsaturated	77	62	46	26	60	30

There are three other types of fat: the 'best', the 'acceptable', and the 'really ugly'. The 'really ugly' fats are potentially the most dangerous. They are vegetable oils that have been heat-treated to make them thicken. These hydrogenated oils or trans fatty acids take on the worst characteristics of saturated fats. So don't use them and avoid foods whose labels list hydrogenated oils or partially hydrogenated oils among their ingredients. Many crackers, cereals, baked goods and fast foods contain these really ugly fats.

So we're avoiding the 'bad' fats and the 'really ugly' fats, but we mustn't eliminate fat entirely from our diet. Fats are absolutely essential to our health as they contain various key elements that are crucial to the digestive process. The 'best' fats are monounsaturated fats and they are found in foods like olives, peanuts, almonds and olive and rapeseed oils. Monounsaturated fats actually have a beneficial effect on cholesterol and are good for your heart. So try to incorporate them into your diet and look for them on food labels. Most manufacturers who use them will say so, because they know it's a key selling point for informed consumers.

Another highly beneficial oil, which is in a category of its own, contains a wonderful ingredient called omega-3. This oil is found in coldwater fish such as salmon and in flax and rapeseed seeds, and it's extremely good for your heart health. 'Acceptable' fats are the polyunsaturated fats because they are cholesterol free. Most vegetable oils, such as corn and sunflower, fall into this category.

By now you must be wondering what causes people to gain weight if it isn't fat. Well, the answer lies in something you've probably never thought of as fattening at all – and that's grain. Have you noticed the multiplying number of grocery store shelves dedicated to products made from flour, corn and rice? Supermarkets now have huge biscuit and snack food sections; whole aisles of cereals; numerous shelves of pastas and noodles; and baskets and baskets of bagels, rolls, muffins and loaves of bread. In 1970 the average North American ate about 135 pounds of grain. By 2000 that figure had risen to nearly *200* pounds! This staggering increase helps explain why over half of British adults are overweight, and why 1 in 5 are considered obese – triple the number 20 years ago! We're definitely eating too much grain, but the other half of the problem is the *type* of grain we're eating, which is generally highly processed. Take flour, for

GRAIN CONSUMPTION (pounds per capita)

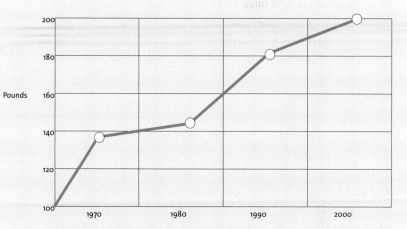

Source: U.S. Department of Agriculture

instance. Today's high-speed flour mills use steel rollers rather than traditional grinding stones to produce an extraordinarily finely ground product. The whole wheat is steamed and scarified by tiny razor-sharp blades to remove the bran and the endosperm. Then the wheat germ and oil are removed because they turn rancid too quickly to last on supermarket shelves. What's left after all that processing is then bleached and marketed as all-purpose flour. This is what almost all the breads, bagels, muffins, cookies, biscuits, cereals and pastas we consume are made of. Even many 'brown' breads are simply artificially coloured white bread.

And it's not just flour that's highly processed nowadays. A hundred years ago most of the food people ate came straight from the farm to the dinner table. Lack of refrigeration and scant knowledge of food chemistry meant that most food remained in its original state. However, advances in science, along with the migration of many women out of the kitchen and into the workforce, led to a revolution in prepared foods. Everything became geared to speed and simplicity of preparation. We now have instant rice and potatoes, as well as entire meals that are ready to eat after just a few minutes in the microwave.

The trouble with all this is that the more a food is processed beyond its natural state, the less processing your body has to do to digest it. And the quicker you digest your food, the sooner you are hungry again and the more you tend to eat. We all know the difference between eating a bowl of old-fashioned, slow-cooking oatmeal and a bowl of sugary cold cereal. The oatmeal stays with you – it 'sticks to your ribs' as my mother used to say – whereas you are looking for your next meal only an hour after eating the bowl of sugary cereal. Our fundamental problem, then, is that we are eating foods that are digested by our bodies too easily. Clearly we can't wind back the clock to simpler times, but we need to somehow slow down the digestive process so we feel hungry less often. How can we do that? Well, we have to eat foods that are *slow-release,* that break down at a *slow and steady rate* in our digestive system, leaving us feeling fuller for longer.

There are two clues to identifying slow-release foods. The first is the amount of fibre in the food. Fibre, in simple terms, provides low-calorie filler. It does double duty, in fact, by literally filling up your stomach so that you feel satiated; and by taking much longer to break down in your body, so the digestive process is slowed and the food stays with you longer. There are two forms of fibre: soluble and insoluble. Soluble fibre is found in foods like oatmeal, beans, barley and citrus fruits, and has been shown to lower blood cholesterol levels. Insoluble fibre is important for normal bowel function and is typically found in whole wheat breads and cereals and most vegetables.

The second tool in identifying slow-release foods is the glycemic index, or G.I., which is the basis of the G.I. Diet and the secret to successful weight management. It was developed by Dr. David Jenkins, a professor of nutrition at the University of Toronto. Early in his career, he became interested in diabetes, a disease that hampers the body's ability to process carbohydrates and sugar (glucose). Sugar therefore stays in the bloodstream instead of going into the body's cells, resulting in hyperglycemia and potentially coma. At the time Dr. Jenkins was beginning his research, carbohydrates were severely restricted in a diabetic's diet because they quickly boost the sugar level in the blood stream. But because the primary role of carbohydrates is to provide the body with energy, diabetics were having to make up the lack of calories through a high-fat diet, which provides energy without boosting sugar levels. Now doctors were in a real quandary: although they were saving diabetics from hyperglycemia, they were accelerating their risk of heart disease.

Dr. Jenkins wondered if all carbohydrates are the same. Are some digested more quickly and as a result raise blood sugar levels faster than others? And are others slow-release, resulting in only a marginal increase in blood sugar? The answer, he discovered, is yes. In 1980, he published an index – the glycemic index –

Sugar	100	Rice (basmati)	58	Apple	38
Baguette	95	Muffin (bran)	56	Cheerios	35
Rice	87	Potatoes (new/boiled)	56	Yoghurt (low fat)	33
Cornflakes	84	Popcorn (light)	55	Fettuccine	32
Potatoes (baked)	84	Orange	44	Beans	31
Doughnut	76	All-Bran	43	Grapefruit	25
Bagel	72	Oatmeal	42	Yoghurt (fat free/no sugar)	14
Raisins	64	Spaghetti	41		
		Tomato	38		

showing the various rates at which carbohydrates break down and release glucose into the bloodstream. The faster the food breaks down, the higher the rating on the index, which sets sugar at 100 and scores all other foods against that number. The chart above contains some examples of G.I. ratings.

By eating only those foods that have a low G.I. rating, diabetics were now able to keep their glucose levels low and avoid hyperglycemia.

As it turns out, the G.I. also has exciting implications for anyone who wishes to lose weight. It has been proven that keeping glucose levels low is the key to permanent weight loss. This is how it works: when you eat a high-G.I. food, your body rapidly converts it into glucose. The glucose dissolves in your bloodstream and spikes its glucose level, giving you that 'sugar high'. The chart on page 13 illustrates the impact of digesting sugar on the level of glucose in your bloodstream compared with kidney beans, which have a low G.I. rating.

G.I. IMPACT ON SUGAR LEVELS

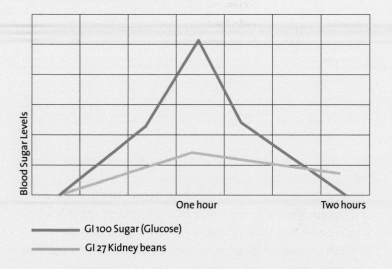

Blood Sugar Levels

One hour   Two hours

— GI 100 Sugar (Glucose)
— GI 27 Kidney beans

As you can see, there is a dramatic difference between the two. What is also apparent from the chart is that after your glucose level spikes, it quickly disappears from your bloodstream, leaving you feeling starved of energy and looking for more fuel. Something most of us experience regularly is the feeling of lethargy that follows an hour or so after a fast-food lunch, which generally consists of high-G.I. foods. The surge of glucose followed by the rapid drain leaves us feeling sluggish and hungry. So what do we do? Around mid-afternoon we look for a quick sugar fix, or snack, to bring us out of the slump. A few cookies or a bag of chips – also high-G.I. foods – cause another rush of glucose, which again disappears a short time later. And so the vicious cycle continues. Eating a diet of high-G.I. foods will obviously make you feel hungry more often and you will end up eating more as a result. Low-G.I. foods, on the other hand, are the tortoise to the high-G.I. foods' hare. They break down in your digestive system at a slow, steady rate. Tortoise-like, they stay the course, making you feel full longer, and consequently, you eat less.

There is a second reason why you should avoid eating high-G.I. foods when you are trying to lose weight. When you experience a rapid spike in your blood sugar, your pancreas releases the hormone insulin. Insulin does two things extremely well. First, it reduces the level of glucose in your bloodstream by diverting it into various body tissues for immediate short-term use or by storing it as fat – which is why glucose disappears so quickly. Second, it inhibits the conversion of body fat back into glucose for the body to burn. This evolutionary feature is a throwback to the days when our ancestors were hunter-gatherers, habitually experiencing times of feast or famine. When food was in abundance, the body stored its surplus as fat to tide it over the days when there wouldn't be much to eat. Insulin was the champion in this process, both helping to accumulate fat and then guarding its depletion.

Today, everything has changed but our stomachs. We don't have to hunt for food anymore – there's a guaranteed supply at the supermarket. But our insulin continues to store fat and keep it intact. As everyone knows, our bodies must be able to access and draw down from our fat cells in order to lose weight. To allow that to happen, you need to do two things. First, you must consume fewer calories than your body needs in order to burn up those fat stores. Now, I hate to bring up calories since we've probably all been driven nearly over the edge with having to count them and perform complex mathematical calculations

Dear Rick,

I am thrilled with my 3½-stone weight loss (in less than four months) and the significant reduction in my blood sugar. Your book has given me renewed hope in getting my weight off, as I have 3½ stones more to go. It is so confidence-building to know that it is not my fault for my morbid obesity these past many years, and I only wish I had known this information years ago. I cannot thank you enough!

Irene

with them. But unfortunately, unless one denies the basic laws of thermodynamics, the equation never changes: consume more calories than you expend and the surplus is stored in the body as fat. That's the inescapable fact. Few diet books today mention calories, but they're there, hidden behind the various rules and suggestions. Don't worry, though, because with *Living the G.I. Diet* you can easily reduce your calorie intake without having to do any calculations and without going hungry – I'll explain how in a moment.

The second thing we must do to enable our bodies to use up its fat cells, is to keep our insulin levels low, which means avoiding high-G.I. foods. Remember the cornflakes, chicken noodle soup, white bread and rice cakes that were mentioned at the beginning of this chapter? Well, you would never lose weight if you ate those foods on a daily basis because they all have high G.I. ratings – they raise your insulin levels to the point where your body won't burn up those fat stores. Instead, you should stick to

Dear Rick,

I lost over 3 stones in just over two months (from 15 stones to 12 stones). No more headaches! My blood pressure is back down from 180/120 to a normal reading – my doctor can't believe the change. This is the best I've felt in years. I weigh less than I did the day I got married sixteen years ago. I'm not hungry between meals with your meal plans and yes, I can indulge once in a while without putting any weight back on.

Many, many thanks,

Joe

low-G.I. foods. Instead of having cornflakes for breakfast, have porridge or homemade muesli. Instead of lunching on chicken noodle soup, enjoy a bowl of homemade lentil soup. Avoid the rice cakes when you need a snack, and have a handful of hazelnuts or almonds instead. It isn't difficult to substitute low-G.I. foods for high-G.I. ones, but by making these changes, your weight will begin to drop. It's that easy. How will you know which foods are high-G.I. and which ones are low? In the next chapter you'll find a comprehensive chart that identifies the foods that will make you fat and those that will allow you to lose weight. Don't expect the foods in the latter category to be limited and boring – there are so many tasty and satisfying choices that you won't even feel as though you are on a diet. And later in this book, Emily Richards will give you many delicious ways to prepare them.

2 The G.i. Diet

Now that you understand the science behind the G.I. Diet, it's time to get down to the nitty gritty. Basically, you need to know what, when and how much to eat to start shedding those extra pounds. Let's begin by addressing the 'what'. As you know from the last chapter, the key to losing weight is to eat foods that have two essential characteristics: a low calorie content and a low G.I. rating. To help you identify those foods, I have developed an easy-to-use reference tool called the G.I. Diet Food Guide.

THE G.I. DIET FOOD GUIDE

This chart lists every food you can think of in one of three categories based on the colours of a traffic light. Foods listed in the red-light or 'stop' category are high-G.I., high-calorie foods that should be avoided. Some of these may surprise you, for example, melba toast, mashed potatoes, turnip and watermelon are all red-light. Your body digests them so quickly that you are hungry again an hour later. Foods in the yellow-light or 'caution' category – for example, sourdough bread, corn and bananas – have moderate G.I. ratings, but they do raise insulin levels to the point where weight loss is not going to happen. Foods in the green-light or 'go ahead' category are the ones that will allow you to lose weight. Chicken, long-grain rice and asparagus are all green-light foods. Eat them and watch your weight drop. After you've had a chance to look over the G.I. Diet Food Guide, we'll talk about how to make it work for you.

	RED	YELLOW	GREEN
BEANS	Baked beans with pork		All beans (tinned or dried)
	Broad		Baked beans (low fat)
	Refried beans		Black-eyed peas
			Chickpeas
			Soybeans
			Split peas
BEVERAGES	Alcoholic drinks*	Diet soft drinks (caffeinated)	Bottled water
	Fruit drinks	Milk (semi-skimmed)	Tonic water
	Milk (whole)	Red wine*	Decaffeinated coffee (with skimmed milk, no sugar)
	Regular coffee	Regular coffee (with skimmed milk, no sugar)	Diet soft drinks (no caffeine)
	Regular soft drinks	Unsweetened fruit juices (see page 24)	Light instant chocolate
	Sweetened juice		Milk (skimmed)
			Tea (with skimmed milk, no sugar)

*In Phase II a glass of wine and the occasional beer may be included

BREADS

Bagels	Pita (whole wheat)	100% stone-ground wholemeal*
Baguette/Croissants	Whole grain breads	Homemade muffins (see p. 167–169)
Cake/Biscuits		Homemade pancakes (see pp. 104 and 106)
Cereal/Granola bars		Whole grain, high-fibre breads (2½ to 3g of fibre per slice)*
Doughnuts		
Scones, crumpets		
Hamburger buns		
Hot dog buns		
Kaiser rolls		
Melba toast		
Muffins		
Pancakes/Waffles		
Pizza		
Stuffing		
Tortillas		
White bread		

* Use a single slice only per serving

	RED	YELLOW	GREEN
CEREALS	All cold cereals except those listed as yellow – or green-light	Shredded Wheat Bran	All-Bran
			Bran Buds
			Fibre First
			High Fibre Bran/Alpen
	Granola		Homemade Muesli (p.115)
	Muesli (commercial)		Oat bran
			Porridge oats (traditional large-flake)
CEREAL GRAINS	Couscous	Corn	Barley
	Millet		Buckwheat
	Rice (short grain, white, instant)		Bulgur
	Rice cakes		Rice (basmati, wild, brown, long grain)
	Croutons		Wheat grain

CONDIMENTS/ SEASONINGS		
Ketchup		Garlic
Mayonnaise		Herbs/Spices
Tartar sauce		Hummus
		Mayonnaise (fat free)
		Mustard
		Soy sauce (low sodium)
		Teriyaki sauce
		Vinegar
		Worcestershire sauce

DAIRY		
Cheese	Cheese (low fat)	Buttermilk
Chocolate milk	Cream cheese (light)	Cheese (fat free)
Cottage cheese (regular)	Ice cream (low fat)	Cottage cheese (low fat or fat free)
Cream	Milk (semi-skimmed)	Fruit yoghurt (fat and sugar free)

RED	YELLOW	GREEN
Cream cheese	Frozen yoghurt (low fat, low sugar)	Ice cream (low fat and no added sugar, e.g. Wall's Too Good to be True)
Milk (whole)	Yoghurt (low fat)	Milk (skimmed)
Sour cream		
Yoghurt (regular)	creme fraiche (low fat)	
Butter	Corn oil	Almonds*
Coconut oil	Mayonnaise (light)	Canola oil*/rapeseed oil
Hard margarine	Most nuts	Flax seed
Lard	Peanut oil	Hazelnuts*
Mayonnaise	Salad dressings (light)	Macadamia nuts*
Palm oil	Sesame oil	Mayonnaise (fat free)
Peanut butter (all varieties)	Soft margarine (non-hydrogenated)	Olive oil*
Salad dressings (regular)	Sunflower oil	Salad dressings (fat free)

FATS AND OILS

*Limit quantity (see serving size on p.30).

Tropical oils	Vegetable oils	Soft margarine (non-hydrogenated, light)*
Vegetable shortening		Vegetable oil sprays

FRUITS – FRESH

Cantaloupe	Apricots (fresh)	Apples
Dates	Bananas	Blackberries
Honeydew melon	Kiwi	Blueberries
Raisins	Mangoes	Cherries
Watermelon	Papaya	Grapefruit
	Pineapple	Grapes
		Lemons
		Oranges (all varieties)
		Peaches/Plums
		Pears
		Raspberries
		Strawberries

*Limit quantity (see serving size on p.30).

	RED	YELLOW	GREEN
FRUITS – BOTTLED, TINNED, FROZEN, DRIED *For baking, it is okay to use a modest amount of dried fruit*	All tinned fruit in syrup Apple sauce containing sugar Most dried fruit*	Dried apricots Dried cranberries Fruit cocktail in juice	Apple sauce (without sugar) Frozen berries Mandarin oranges Peaches in juice or water Pears in juice or water
FRUIT JUICES *Whenever possible eat the fruit rather than drink its juice*	Fruit drinks Sweetened juices Prune Watermelon	Apple (unsweetened) Cranberry (unsweetened) Grapefruit (unsweetened) Orange (unsweetened) Pear (unsweetened) Pineapple (unsweetened)	
MEAT, POULTRY, FISH, EGGS AND SOY *Avoid breaded or battered seafood*	Minced beef (more than 10% fat) Hamburgers	Minced beef (lean) Lamb (lean cuts)	All seafood, fresh, frozen or tinned*** Back bacon

Hot dogs	Pork (lean cuts)	Beef (lean cuts)
Processed meats	Turkey bacon	Chicken breast (skinless)
Regular bacon	Whole omega-3 eggs (e.g. Columbus)	Minced beef (extra lean)
Sausages		Lean deli ham
Whole regular eggs		Egg whites
		Quorn**
Sushi (it's the rice)		Sashimi
		Soy/whey protein powder
		Tofu
		Turkey breast (skinless)
		Veal
All tinned pastas		Capellini
Gnocchi		Fettuccine
Macaroni and cheese		Macaroni
Noodles (tinned or instant)		Penne
Pasta filled with with cheese or meat		Spaghetti/Linguine
		Vermicelli

PASTA*

*Try to use wholemeal or protein-enriched pasta (see serving size on p.30).

** Possible health risk (see www.cspinet.org).

	RED	YELLOW	GREEN
PASTA SAUCES	Alfredo	Sauces with vegetables (no added sugar)	Light sauces with vegetables (no added sugar)
	Sauces with added meat or cheese		
	Sauces with added sugar or sucrose		
SNACKS *Limit quantity (see serving size on p.30)*	Bagels	Bananas	Almonds*
	Bread	Dark chocolate (70% cocoa)*	Apple sauce (unsweetened)
	Chocolates and sweets	Ice cream (low fat)	Tinned peaches/pears in juice or water
	Cookies	Most nuts*	Cottage cheese (1% or fat free)
	Biscuits	Popcorn (light, microwaveable)	Food bars (see p.176)
	Doughnuts		Fruit yoghurt (fat and sugar free)
	French fries		Ice cream (low fat and no added sugar, e.g. Wall's Too Good to be True)
	Ice cream		

Hazelnuts*		Jell-O (all varieties)
Homemade muffins (p.167)		Muffins (commercial)
Most fresh fruit		Popcorn (regular)
Most fresh vegetables		Crisps/Pretzels
Soy nuts*		Raisins
Snack recipes starting on p.164		Rice cakes
		Sorbet
		Tortilla chips
		Mixed dried fruit and nuts

SOUPS

All homemade soups made with green-light ingredients.	Tinned chicken noodle	All cream-based soups
Chunky bean and vegetable soups (e.g. Baxter's Healthy Choice)	Tinned lentil	Tinned black bean
	Tinned tomato	Tinned green pea
		Puréed vegetable
		Tinned split pea

	RED	YELLOW	GREEN
SUGAR AND SWEETENERS** ***See sweeteners on p.182*	Corn syrup Glucose Honey Molasses Sugar (all types) Treacle	Fructose	Aspartame Hermesetas Gold Splenda Stevia
VEGETABLES	Broad beans French fries Hash browns Parsnips Potatoes (instant) Potatoes (mashed or baked) Swede Turnip	Artichokes Beets Corn Avocado (¼ per serving) Potatoes (boiled) Pumpkin Squash Sweet potatoes Yams	Arugula Asparagus Aubergine Beans (green/runner) Bell peppers/ Capsicums Broccoli Brussels sprouts Cabbage Carrots

Cauliflower

Celery

Chilli peppers

Collard greens

Courgettes

Cucumbers

Kale

Lettuce (all varieties)

Leeks

Mangetouts

Mushrooms

Olives*

Onions

Peas

Pickles

Potatoes (boiled new)*

Spinach

Swiss chard

Sugar snap

Radishes

Tomatoes

* Limit quantity (see serving size on p.30)

SERVINGS AND PORTIONS

The G.I. Diet Food Guide makes choosing the right foods for your new eating plan easy. But how much of them should you eat and when? First of all, this isn't a deprivation diet. For the most part, you can have as much of the green-light foods as you like. There are only a few exceptions, which have a higher G.I. rating or calorie content than others. I've listed them along with their recommended serving sizes below.

Green-light breads (which have at least 2½ to 3 grams of fibre per slice)	1 slice
Green-light cereals	120g (4oz)
Green-light nuts	8 to 10
Margarine (non-hydrogenated, light)	2 teaspoons
Meat, fish, poultry	120g (4oz) (about the size of a pack of cards)
Olive/rapeseed oil	1 teaspoon
Olives	4 to 5
Pasta	40g (1½oz) uncooked
Potatoes (boiled new)	2 to 3
Rice (basmati, brown, long grain)	50g (1¾oz) uncooked
PHASE II	
Chocolate (70% cocoa)	2 squares
Red wine	1 125ml (5fl oz) glass

Some readers have asked me if it's okay to eat twelve apples a day or an entire tub of cottage cheese at a sitting! I don't recommend that you go overboard on quantities of anything.

Moderation is key. It's also important that you spread your daily calorie intake evenly throughout the day. If your digestive system is busy processing food and steadily supplying energy to your brain, you won't be looking for high-calorie snacks. I know that many people make a habit of skipping breakfast in the morning, but this is a big mistake. People who miss breakfast leave their stomachs empty from dinner to lunch the next day, often more than sixteen hours! No wonder they overeat at lunch and then look for a sugar fix mid-afternoon as they run out of steam. Always eat three meals – breakfast, lunch and dinner – as well as three snacks – one mid-morning, one mid-afternoon and one before bed – each day. And try to consume approximately the same amount of calories at each principal meal. If you eat a tiny breakfast and then a tiny lunch, you'll feel so hungry by dinner time that you won't be able to stop yourself from overeating.

As well, each meal should contain some vegetables or fruit, some protein and some type of whole grain food. Fruits, vegetables and grains are all carbohydrates, which are the primary source of energy for your body. They are rich in fibre, vitamins and minerals, including antioxidants, which we now believe play a critical role in protecting against disease – especially heart disease and cancer. That's one of the reasons why high-protein diets, which unfortunately have become quite popular in recent years, are so harmful to your long-term health. They prescribe eating a great deal of animal protein, which is high in saturated fat, while severely cutting back on carbohydrates. This causes ketosis, a dangerous electrolyte imbalance and an acid build-up in the blood that can lead to kidney damage, kidney stones and osteoporosis. Side effects include fatigue, headache, nausea, dizziness and bad breath. By minimizing the amount of vegetables, fruits, whole grains and legumes you consume, you deprive your body of essential vitamins and minerals.

With that in mind, vegetables and fruit, most of which are low-calorie and low-G.I., form the base of the G.I. Diet. Now, most offical sources have traditionally suggested that grains should be the largest component of your diet, followed by vegetables and fruit. But by giving grains priority, they are promoting the leading cause of overweight and obesity. Recently, the Mayo Clinic, one of the world's leading medical research centres, has begun to promote vegetables and fruits as the basis of a healthy diet, rather than grains, which is exactly what the G.I. Diet recommends.

Protein is another essential part of your diet. One-half of your dry body weight is made up of protein, i.e., your muscles, organs, skin and hair, and protein is required to build and repair body tissue. It is also much more effective than carbohydrates or fat in satisfying hunger. It acts as a brake in the digestive process and will make you feel fuller longer as well as more alert. So please include some protein in every single meal. Too often we grab a hasty breakfast of coffee and toast – a protein-free meal. Lunch is sometimes not much better: a bowl of pasta with a few slivers of chicken. And a typical afternoon snack of a biscuit, piece of fruit or muffin contains not a gram of protein. Generally, it's not until dinner that we eat protein, usually our entire daily recommended allowance plus some extra. But because protein is a critical brain food, providing amino acids for the neurotransmitters that relay messages in the brain, it would be

TRADITIONAL   **GI DIET**

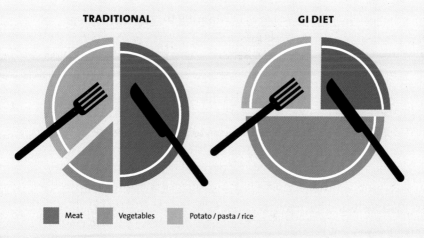

■ Meat   ■ Vegetables   ■ Potato / pasta / rice

better to load up on it earlier in the day. That would give you an alert and active mind for your daily activities. The best solution, however, as I've said, is to spread your protein consumption throughout the day to keep you on the ball and feeling full. Choose low-fat proteins such as lean or low-fat meats that have been trimmed of any visible fat; skinless poultry; fresh, frozen or tinned fish (but not the kind that's coated in batter, which is invariably high in fat); shellfish; beans; low-fat dairy products like skimmed milk (believe it or not, after a couple of weeks of drinking it, it tastes just like semi-skimmed), low-fat yoghurt without sugar, and low-fat cottage cheese; egg whites; and tofu.

An easy way to visualize the portion sizes you should be consuming is to imagine your plate divided into three sections. Half the plate should be covered with vegetables and fruit. One of the sources of protein listed above should occupy one quarter of the plate, and the last quarter should be filled with a green-light type of rice, pasta or potato. Above is a diagram of what your green-light dinner plate should look like.

What to Have for Breakfast

My favourite breakfast of all time is good old-fashioned porridge oats. Not only is it low-G.I. and low-calorie, but it also lowers cholesterol. Be sure to use the large-flake variety and not the one-minute or instant oats, which have been processed. Porridge will stay with you all morning and it is easy to prepare, especially in the microwave. You can also endlessly vary the flavour by adding non-fat, sugar-free, fruit-flavoured yoghurt; unsweetened apple sauce/purée, or fruit. Emily has included some fabulous breakfast ideas, starting on page 100. To make your regular breakfasts green-light, here are some general guidelines to follow.

Coffee

The principal problem with coffee is its caffeine content. There is growing evidence to suggest that caffeine causes your body to produce high levels of insulin – which is the last thing we want. That's why I recommend you drink only decaffeinated coffee when you are trying to lose weight. If you simply can't face the day without a cup of java, caffeine intact, then please, go ahead and have it. But don't add sugar – use a sweetener instead – and add only semi-skimmed or skimmed milk. I have received so many e-mails from readers who feel that caffeine deprivation is a definite deal breaker. If you follow the other principles of the G.I. Diet, you can have your morning cup of coffee and still reach your weight-loss target.

Dear Rick,

Like many others, I'm sure, I've tried different approaches
to losing weight and eating healthier, but I still find myself
engaged in the same battle, month after month. I used to
blame it on age. I'm getting older, getting bigger, losing the
hair on my head just to watch it grow on my back – now that's
a pretty picture. I'd better stop. After reading your book, I
understand and feel better about a whole lot of things.

Thank God for me because I love porridge and eat it every
morning. . . . I believe, therefore I'm doing it. I eat better, I
exercise more and it won't be long before I lose the remaining
eleven pounds. I recently went home for Mother's Day. My
sister-in-law said, 'Dan, I find it so funny that before, you
would eat like a bird, and now you say you are following a diet,
but you haven't stopped eating.' She was right and it is funny
because I am losing weight and I feel great. I'm going to my
grandmother's this weekend. I'm sure she'll get a good laugh
when I walk in with my bag of oatmeal.

Thanks, you've made a difference.

Dan

Juice/Fruit

Always eat the fruit rather than drink its juice. Juice is a processed product that is more rapidly digested than the parent fruit. To illustrate the point, diabetics who run into an insulin crisis and are in a state of hypoglycemia (low blood sugar) are usually given orange juice because it's the fastest way to get glucose into the bloodstream. A glass of juice has 2½ times the calories of a fresh whole orange.

Cereals

Aside from porridge, go for the high-fibre products that have at least 10 grams of fibre per serving. Oat bran is also excellent. Though these cereals are not much fun in themselves, you can liven them up with fresh or tinned fruit, nuts, and non-fat, sugar-free, fruit-flavoured yoghurt. You can also add sweetener (though stay away from sugar).

Toast

Always use bread that has at least 2½ to 3 grams of fibre per slice. Most of the nutrient content labels on breads list fibre for a two-slice serving, which should be 5 to 6 grams. Remember, however, that a green-light serving is only *one slice* per meal. A good choice of bread is 100% stone-ground wholemeal. 'Stone-ground' means the flour has been ground with stones rather than steel rollers, resulting in a coarser grind and a lower G.I. rating.

Spreads

Do not use butter. The latest premium brands of non-hydrogenated soft margarine are acceptable and the light versions even more so, but still use them sparingly. In fruit

spreads, look for the 'extra fruit/sugar-reduced' versions.
These taste terrific and are remarkably low in calories.

Eggs

In Phase I use egg whites where possible. Otherwise, use omega-3 whole eggs (e.g. Columbus) but limit the number to seven per week. Unless you have a medical cholesterol problem, you may eat as many as you wish in Phase II.

Bacon

Sorry, but regular bacon is a red-light food. Acceptable alternatives are Canadian back bacon, turkey bacon and lean ham.

Dairy

Low-fat dairy products are a great source of protein in the morning. I always have a glass of skimmed milk with breakfast. Try moving down from semi-skimmed to skimmed in stages. I find that semi-skimmed tastes like cream now!

Low- or non-fat yogurts that do not contain sugar, and low-fat or fat-free cottage cheese and cream cheese are also excellent sources of protein. Try to stay away from other cheeses, though, since they are generally high in saturated fat.

WHAT TO HAVE FOR LUNCH

Since most of us spend the lunch hour away from home, either at work or school, we tend to have two options for the midday meal: (1) we can take a packed lunch, or (2) we can eat at a restaurant. In both cases, eating the green-light way is definitely doable – but there are some important guidelines to keep in mind.

Packed lunches

This is really the best option for the G.I. dieter. When you pack your own lunch, you can be sure that all the ingredients used are green-light. Here are some tips for turning your brown-bag into a green-light bag.

Sandwiches

This popular lunchtime mainstay is usually high-G.I. and high-calorie. But there are several things you can do to make your sandwich green-light. First, use one slice of 100% stone-ground wholemeal or other high-fibre bread. Spread on some mustard or hummus (no butter or margarine) and top with 4 ounces of lean deli ham, chicken, turkey or fish. Add at least three vegetables, such as lettuce, tomato, cucumber or green pepper. And do not top the sandwich with another slice of bread, simply eat it open-faced. Avoid egg- and tuna-salad sandwiches that are made with fattening mayonnaise.

Salads

Salads are almost always green-light but are often short on protein. Add in chickpeas or other types of beans, or 120g (4oz) of tuna, salmon, tofu, skinless, cooked chicken breast or other lean meat. Also watch the dressing. Use only low-fat or fat-free versions. There are some great salad recipes starting on page 117.

Soups

In general, commercially tinned soups have a relatively high G.I. rating because of the necessary high temperatures used in the canning process. There are a few green-light brands, such as Baxter's Healthy Choice. Homemade soups made with green-light ingredients are the best option, and Emily has provided some recipes starting on page 110. Beware of all cream-based or puréed vegetable soups, since they are high in fat and heavily processed.

Pasta

The thing to watch out for here is quantity. Your pasta dish should contain only 40g (1¹⁄₃oz) of cooked, preferably wholemeal pasta, as well as 90g (3oz) of vegetables, 60ml (2fl oz) of light pasta sauce, and 4 ounces of chicken or lean deli meat.

Cottage Cheese and Fruit

A fast and easy lunch to take to work is cottage cheese and fruit. Pack 240g (8oz) of low-fat or fat-free cottage cheese and 150-210g (5–7oz) of green-light fruit.

Dessert

Always have some fresh fruit for dessert. Pass on other sweet things at lunch time.

Lunching Out

I have provided a handy page of tips for eating out at restaurants on page 183. Basically, all you have to do is order an entrée that includes a low-fat source of protein, such as chicken or fish, and vegetables. Ask for extra vegetables in lieu of potatoes or rice, since restaurants tend to serve the red-light versions. Eating at a fast-food outlet, however, is another story. Because fast food is loaded with saturated fat and calories, with rarely a gram of fibre in sight, it is usually a good idea to avoid it. It's true that some major fast-food chains have recently started offering lower-fat options, but by going into the restaurant, you are walking into a den of temptation, surrounded by people scarfing down their usual fare of dietary disasters. If your alternatives are limited, however, here are some guidelines for navigating this gastronomic minefield.

Burgers
Dispose of the top of the bun and don't order cheese or bacon. Keep it as simple as possible.

Fries
DON'T. A medium order of McDonald's fries contains 17 grams of fat (mostly saturated), about 50 per cent of your total daily allowance.

Milkshakes
DON'T. The saturated fat and calorie levels are unbelievable.

Wraps
An increasingly popular alternative to the traditional sandwich is a wrap. Request a wholemeal pita if available and ask that it be split in half.

Submarines

An open-faced whole wheat sub is the basis of a reasonable green-light meal. Avoid cheese and mayonnaise unless they're low fat.

Fish or shellfish

Both are excellent choices providing there's no batter or breaded coating.

Chinese

My best advice is to steer clear of Chinese restaurants when trying to lose weight. The rice is a problem, because it is usually the high-G.I., glutinous kind that tends to stick together. The sauces, especially the sweet and sour ones, are high in sugar and the noodles are also high G.I.

WHAT TO SNACK ON

I can't stress enough how important it is to have three snacks every day. Snacks play a critical role between meals by giving you a boost when you most need it. Choose fruit; fat-free, sugar-free yoghurt; low-fat or fat-free cottage cheese; raw vegetables, nuts, and Emily's snack recipes on pages 164 to 169. Watch out for other products that claim to be fat- and sugar-free, such as pudding. Unfortunately these products are usually made with highly processed grain and are red-light. You might also want to look into food bars. Choose 50- to 65-gram bars that have around 200 calories each with 20 to 30 grams of carbohydrates, 12 to 15 grams of protein and 5 grams of fat. In the UK these are sometimes hard to find. Check your local sports equipment or health-food shop. Most so-called nutrition bars found in supermarkets are high-G.I., high-calorie, and contain lots of quick-fix carbs. Check labels carefully.

WHAT TO HAVE FOR DINNER

The typical British dinner comprises three things: meat or fish; potato, pasta or rice; and vegetables. Together, these foods provide an assortment of carbohydrates, proteins and fats, along with other minerals and vitamins essential to our health.

Meat/Fish

Most meats contain saturated fat, so it's important to buy lean cuts and trim off all the visible fat. Chicken and turkey are excellent choices *provided all the skin is removed*. And fish and shellfish (not breaded) are also wonderful. In terms of quantity, the best measure for meat or fish is your palm. The portion should fit into the palm of your hand and be about as thick. Another good visual is a pack of cards.

Potatoes

The G.I. ratings of potatoes vary from high to moderate, depending on how they are cooked. Boiled new potatoes are the only kind you should eat, two or three at a sitting. Baked, mashed and fried potatoes are all red-light.

Pasta

Though most pastas have a moderate G.I. rating and are low in fat, they have become a villain in weight control. That's because we tend to eat too much of it. Italians quite rightly view pasta as an appetizer or side dish, while we make it a main course with sauce and a few slivers of meat. Pasta should only make up a quarter of your meal (about 40g [1¹⁄₃oz] uncooked). Use whole wheat or protein- enriched pasta and stay away from cream-based sauces.

Rice

Rice also has a broad G.I. range. The low ones are basmati, wild, brown and long-grain because they contain a starch, amylose, that breaks down more slowly than that of other rices. Serving size is critical, too. Allow 50 grams (1²⁄₃oz) of dry rice per serving.

Vegetables/Salad

Eat green-light vegetables and salad to your heart's content. Serve two or three varieties of vegetables at every dinner as well as a salad.

Desserts

There is a broad range of low-G.I., low-calorie desserts that taste great and are good for you. Virtually any fruit qualifies and there's always low-fat, sugar-free ice cream. And wait till you try Emily's Baked Chocolate Mousse (page 172) and Pecan Brownies (page 174)!

Beverages

We all know that we are supposed to drink eight glasses of fluids per day. Personally, I find this a bit steep. But I do try to drink a glass of water before each meal and snack. Other than to stay hydrated, I do this for two reasons: one, having your stomach partly filled with liquid before the meal means you will feel full more quickly, thus reducing the temptation to overeat; two, you won't be tempted to wash down your food before it's been sufficiently chewed.

Water is definitely the best beverage choice because it doesn't contain any calories. Liquids don't seem to trip our satiety mechanisms, so it's a waste, really, to take in calories through them. Alcohol especially is a disaster for weight control because it is easily metabolized by the body, resulting in increased insulin production – so try to avoid it. It is also wise to stay away from fruit and vegetable juices, which we digest rapidly. If water is too boring for you, there are a number of no-cal or low-cal beverages to choose from.

Coffee

If you can, it's best to stick with decaffeinated coffee (see page 32). Never add sugar and use only semi-skimmed or skimmed milk.

Tea

Both black and green teas have considerably less caffeine than coffee and also contain antioxidants that are beneficial to your heart health. Two cups of tea have the same amount of antioxidants as seven cups of orange juice or twenty of apple juice! So tea in moderation is fine, but use a sweetener if you normally add sugar, and skimmed milk. Herbal teas are also a good choice, though they do not contain the antioxidants that black and green teas have.

Soft Drinks

Most soft drinks are high in both sugar and caffeine, and are therefore red-light. Instead, opt for diet soft drinks that do not contain caffeine.

Skimmed milk

Personally, my favourite beverage is skimmed milk. It's non-fat, and since most lunches tend to be a bit protein deficient, drinking skimmed milk is a good way of making up for some of the shortfall.

Soy Milk

Soy milk can be an excellent choice, but buyer beware: most soy beverages are not only high in fat, but also have added sugar. Look for soy milk that is non-fat or low-fat, that has no flavouring like vanilla or chocolate and that has no added sugar.

Vegetarians

If you are a non-meat eater and need to lose weight, the G.I. Diet is the programme for you. All you have to do is continue to substitute vegetable protein for animal protein – something you've been doing all along. However, because most vegetable protein sources, such as beans, are encased in fibre, your digestive system may not be getting the maximum protein benefit. So try to add some easily digestible protein boosters like tofu and soy protein powder to your meals.

Okay, you now know what, when and how much to eat and drink to start shedding those pounds! In the next chapter, I'll outline the steps for getting started on the G.I. Diet.

3 Getting Started in Phase I

The G.I. Diet consists of two phases, and the first, Phase I, is really the most exciting. This is the weight-loss portion of the diet, when you're putting your newly acquired knowledge into practice, developing healthier eating habits, trying new recipes, watching your waistline diminish and feeling more energized. Once you have achieved your weight-loss goal, you enter Phase II – a heady moment. At this point all you have to do is maintain your new svelte frame, and perhaps buy some new clothes. Ready? Here are the essential first steps for launching yourself into Phase I.

STEP 1: SET THE GOAL

Before you do anything else, get your vital statistics on record. I can't think of a greater motivator than measuring your progress as the pounds drop off. On page 185, you will find a log sheet to record your weekly progress. Always weigh yourself at the same time of day, because a meal or bowel movement can throw off your weight by a couple of pounds. First thing in the morning, before you eat breakfast, is a good time. Another measurement that is important to know is your waist circumference. It indicates your level of abdominal fat, which is significant to your health, especially your heart health. A woman's health is at risk if her waist circumference is 32 inches or more, and a man's is at risk if his is 37 inches or more. A measurement of 35 inches plus for women and 40 inches plus for men puts you in the high-risk category for heart attack and stroke. People with a high level of abdominal fat, whom doctors describe as apple-shaped, have a much higher chance of developing cardiovascular disease and Type 2 diabetes.

To measure your waist, take a measuring tape and wrap it around your natural waistline just above the navel. Don't be tempted to suck your stomach in! Just stand in a relaxed position and keep the measuring tape from cutting into your flesh. Now record your weight and waist measurement on the log sheet. I've added a Comments column so that you can also note how you're feeling, or any unusual events in the past week that might have some bearing on your progress. (Readers have asked for additional log sheets. I suggest you photocopy some extra copies before you start.)

Now that you know what your current weight and waist measurement are, you should set your weight-loss target. How much do you want to lose? The best method for determining this is the Body Mass Index, or BMI. It is the only internationally recognized standard for measuring body fat – which is the only part of you that we're interested in reducing. The BMI table on pages 48 to 49 is very simple to use. Just find your height in the chart in the horizontal column across the top and go down the table until you reach your weight. Where they intersect is your BMI, which is a pretty accurate estimate of the proportion of body fat you're carrying – unless you are under 5'0", are elderly or overly muscled (and you really have to be a dedicated bodybuilder to qualify). If any of these characteristics apply to you, then these numbers, in all probability, do not.

The ideal BMI is between 20 and 25. This range is quite generous, however, and your target BMI should be toward the lower end, preferably around 22. BMI values under 18.5 are considered underweight, while those between 25.0 and 29.0 are classified

WEIGHT				HEIGHT																		
BRITISH		US		FT INS	4'6"	4'8"	4'10"	5'0"	5'2"	5'3"	5'4"	5'5"	5'6"	5'7"	5'8"	5'9"	5'10"	5'11"	6'0"	6'2"	6'4"	6'6"	6'8"
STONES	LBS	POUNDS	KILOS	CM	137	142	147	152	157	160	163	165	168	170	173	175	178	180	183	188	193	198	203
6	7	91	41		22.0	20.4	19.0	17.8	16.6	16.1	15.6	15.1	14.7	14.3	13.8	13.4	13.1	12.7	12.3	11.7	11.1	10.5	10.0
6	10	94	43		22.7	21.1	19.6	18.4	17.2	16.7	16.1	15.6	15.2	14.7	14.3	13.9	13.5	13.1	12.7	12.1	11.4	10.9	10.3
7	0	98	44		23.7	22.0	20.5	19.1	17.9	17.4	16.8	16.3	15.8	15.3	14.9	14.5	14.1	13.7	13.3	12.6	11.9	11.3	10.8
7	3	101	46		24.4	22.6	21.1	19.7	18.5	17.9	17.3	16.8	16.3	15.8	15.4	14.9	14.5	14.1	13.7	13.0	12.3	11.7	11.1
7	7	105	48		25.4	23.5	21.9	20.5	19.2	18.6	18.0	17.5	16.9	16.4	16.0	15.5	15.1	14.6	14.2	13.5	12.8	12.1	11.5
7	10	108	49		26.1	24.2	22.6	21.1	19.8	19.1	18.5	18.0	17.4	16.9	16.4	15.9	15.5	15.1	14.6	13.9	13.1	12.5	11.9
8	0	112	51		27.1	25.1	23.4	21.9	20.5	19.8	19.2	18.6	18.1	17.5	17.0	16.5	16.1	15.6	15.2	14.4	13.6	12.9	12.3
8	3	115	52		27.8	25.8	24.0	22.5	21.0	20.4	19.7	19.1	18.6	18.0	17.5	17.0	16.5	16.0	15.6	14.8	14.0	13.3	12.6
8	7	119	54		28.8	26.7	24.9	23.2	21.8	21.1	20.4	19.8	19.2	18.6	18.1	17.6	17.1	16.6	16.1	15.3	14.5	13.8	13.1
8	10	122	55		29.5	27.4	25.5	23.8	22.3	21.6	20.9	20.3	19.7	19.1	18.5	18.0	17.5	17.0	16.5	15.7	14.9	14.1	13.4
9	3	129	59		31.2	28.9	27.0	25.2	23.6	22.9	22.1	21.5	20.8	20.2	19.6	19.0	18.5	18.0	17.5	16.6	15.7	14.9	14.2
9	7	133	60		32.1	29.8	27.8	26.0	24.3	23.6	22.9	22.1	21.5	20.8	20.2	19.6	19.1	18.5	18.0	17.1	16.2	15.4	14.6
9	10	136	62		32.9	30.5	28.4	26.6	24.9	24.1	23.3	22.6	22.0	21.3	20.7	20.1	19.5	19.0	18.4	17.5	16.6	15.7	14.9
10	0	140	64		33.8	31.4	29.3	27.3	25.6	24.8	24.0	23.3	22.6	21.9	21.3	20.7	20.1	19.5	19.0	18.0	17.0	16.2	15.4
10	3	143	65		34.6	32.1	29.9	27.9	26.2	25.3	24.5	23.8	23.1	22.4	21.7	21.1	20.5	19.9	19.4	18.4	17.4	16.5	15.7
10	7	147	67		35.5	33.0	30.7	28.7	26.9	26.0	25.2	24.5	23.7	23.0	22.4	21.7	21.1	20.5	19.9	18.9	17.9	17.0	16.1
10	10	150	68		36.3	33.6	31.3	29.3	27.4	26.6	25.7	25.0	24.2	23.5	22.8	22.2	21.5	20.9	20.3	19.3	18.3	17.3	16.5
11	0	154	70		37.2	34.5	32.2	30.1	28.2	27.3	26.4	25.6	24.9	24.1	23.4	22.7	22.1	21.5	20.9	19.8	18.7	17.8	16.9
11	3	157	71		37.9	35.2	32.8	30.7	28.7	27.8	26.9	26.1	25.3	24.6	23.9	23.2	22.5	21.9	21.3	20.2	19.1	18.1	17.2
11	7	161	73		38.9	36.1	33.6	31.4	29.4	28.5	27.6	26.8	26.0	25.2	24.5	23.8	23.1	22.5	21.8	20.7	19.6	18.6	17.7
11	10	164	74		39.6	36.8	34.3	32.0	30.0	29.1	28.2	27.3	26.5	25.7	24.9	24.2	23.5	22.9	22.2	21.1	20.0	19.0	18.0
12	0	168	76		40.6	37.7	35.1	32.8	30.7	29.8	28.8	28.0	27.1	26.3	25.5	24.8	24.1	23.4	22.8	21.6	20.4	19.4	18.5
12	3	171	78		41.3	38.3	35.7	33.4	31.3	30.7	29.4	28.5	27.6	26.8	26.0	25.3	24.5	23.8	23.2	22.0	20.8	19.8	18.8
12	7	175	79		42.3	39.2	36.6	34.2	32.0	31.0	30.0	29.1	28.2	27.4	26.6	25.8	25.1	24.4	23.7	22.5	21.3	20.2	19.2

12	10	178	81	19.6	20.6	21.7	22.9	24.1	24.8	25.5	26.3	27.1	27.9	28.7	29.6	30.6	31.5	32.6	34.8	37.2	39.9	43.0
13	0	182	83	20.0	21.0	22.2	23.4	24.7	25.4	26.1	26.9	27.7	28.5	29.4	30.3	31.2	32.2	33.3	35.5	38.0	40.8	44.0
13	3	185	84	20.3	21.4	22.5	23.8	25.1	25.8	26.5	27.3	28.1	29.0	29.9	30.8	31.8	32.8	33.8	36.1	38.7	41.5	44.7
13	7	189	86	20.8	21.8	23.0	24.3	25.6	26.4	27.1	27.9	28.7	29.6	30.5	31.5	32.4	33.5	34.6	36.9	39.5	42.4	45.7
13	10	192	87	21.1	22.2	23.4	24.7	26.0	26.8	27.5	28.4	29.2	30.1	31.0	31.9	33.0	34.0	35.1	37.5	40.1	43.0	46.4
13	0	196	89	21.5	22.6	23.9	25.2	26.6	27.3	28.1	28.9	29.8	30.7	31.6	32.6	33.6	34.7	35.8	38.3	41.0	43.9	47.4
14	3	199	90	21.9	23.0	24.2	25.5	27.0	27.8	28.6	29.4	30.3	31.2	32.1	33.1	34.2	35.3	36.4	38.9	41.6	44.6	48.1
14	7	203	92	22.3	23.5	24.7	26.1	27.5	28.3	29.1	30.0	30.9	31.8	32.8	33.8	34.8	36.0	37.1	39.6	42.4	45.5	49.1
14	10	206	93	22.6	23.8	25.1	26.4	27.9	28.7	29.6	30.4	31.3	32.3	33.2	34.3	35.4	36.5	37.7	40.2	43.1	46.2	49.8
15	0	210	95	23.1	24.3	25.6	27.0	28.5	29.3	30.1	31.0	31.9	32.9	33.9	34.9	36.0	37.2	38.4	41.0	43.9	47.1	50.8
15	3	213	97	23.4	24.6	25.9	27.3	28.9	29.7	30.6	31.5	32.4	33.4	34.4	35.4	36.6	37.7	39.0	41.6	44.5	47.8	51.5
15	7	217	98	23.8	25.1	26.4	27.9	29.4	30.3	31.1	32.0	33.0	34.0	35.0	36.1	37.2	38.4	39.7	42.4	45.4	48.6	52.4
15	10	220	100	24.2	25.4	26.8	28.2	29.8	30.7	31.6	32.5	33.5	34.5	35.5	36.6	37.8	39.0	40.2	43.0	46.0	49.3	53.2
16	0	224	102	24.6	25.9	27.3	28.8	30.4	31.2	32.1	33.1	34.1	35.1	36.2	37.3	38.4	39.7	41.0	43.7	46.8	50.2	54.1
16	3	227	103	24.9	26.2	27.6	29.1	30.8	31.7	32.6	33.5	34.5	35.6	36.6	37.8	39.0	40.2	41.5	44.3	47.4	50.9	54.9
16	7	231	105	25.4	26.7	28.1	29.7	31.3	32.2	33.1	34.1	35.1	36.2	37.3	38.4	39.7	40.9	42.2	45.1	48.3	51.8	55.8
16	10	234	106	25.7	27.0	28.5	30.0	31.7	32.6	33.6	34.6	35.6	36.6	37.8	38.9	40.2	41.5	42.8	45.7	48.9	52.5	56.6
17	0	238	108	26.1	27.5	29.0	30.6	32.3	33.2	34.1	35.1	36.2	37.3	38.4	39.6	40.9	42.2	43.5	46.5	49.7	53.4	57.5
17	7	245	111	26.9	28.3	29.8	31.4	33.2	34.1	35.1	36.1	37.2	38.3	39.6	40.7	42.0	43.3	44.8	47.8	51.2	54.9	59.0
18	0	252	114	27.6	29.1	30.5	32.3	34.1	35.1	36.1	37.2	38.3	39.4	40.6	41.9	43.2	44.6	46.0	49.2	52.6	56.4	60.7
18	7	259	117	28.4	29.9	31.5	33.2	35.1	36.1	37.1	38.2	39.3	40.5	41.8	43.0	44.4	45.8	47.3	50.9	54.1	58.0	62.4
19	0	266	120	29.2	30.7	32.3	34.1	36.0	37.0	38.1	39.2	40.4	41.6	42.9	44.2	45.6	47.1	48.6	51.9	55.5	59.6	64.1
19	7	273	123	29.9	31.5	33.2	35.0	37.0	38.1	39.1	40.3	41.5	42.7	44.0	45.4	46.8	48.3	49.9	53.3	57.0	61.2	65.8
20	0	280	126	30.7	32.3	34.0	35.9	37.9	39.0	40.1	41.3	42.5	43.8	45.1	46.5	48.0	49.5	51.2	54.6	58.5	62.7	67.5

as overweight. BMI values of 30.0 and over are considered obese. Let's look at an example. If Sharon is 5'6" and weighs 11½ stones, her BMI is 26, which is 4 notches above her target BMI of 22. This means that Sharon has to lose 1 stone 11lb in order to bring her to her 22 BMI goal of 9 stones 10lb.

Generally it will take between three and six months to achieve your BMI target. How do I figure that? Well, a pound of fat contains around 3,600 calories. To lose that pound in one week, you must reduce your caloric intake by around 500 calories per day (500 x 7 = 3,500 calories). So if you want to lose twenty pounds, it will take twenty weeks. If that seems like a long time to you, think of it in terms of the rest of your life. What's less than half a year compared with the many, many years you'll spend afterwards with a slim, healthy body? This isn't a fad diet – fad diets don't work. The G.I. Diet is a wholesome, realistic, surefire route to permanent weight loss, and you can do it!

For those of you who have a significant amount of weight to lose, there is good news. The heavier you are, the greater your weight loss will be. It is not unusual for 'big people' to lose an average of 2–3lb a week during Phase I. Let's move on to step 2.

STEP 2: CLEAR OUT THE CUPBOARDS

At this point, your kitchen cupboard and refrigerator still probably contain some of the foods that are listed in the red-light column of the G.I. Diet Food Guide. Now how are you going to reach your goal with all this temptation at your fingertips? Give yourself a break and do something radical: clear out your pantry, fridge and freezer of all red- and yellow-light products. If the thought of throwing them in the garbage makes you blanch, donate the tinned foods and other non-perishables to the local food bank and give the rest to neighbours, your children away at university or anyone you know who doesn't happen to live in your house. This does not mean you will be depriving the non-dieters in your family – this is a healthy way of eating for everyone. You're doing them a service!

STEP 3: GO SHOPPING

After you've enjoyed a good meal – and you're not remotely hungry – head over to the local grocery store and stock up on green-light foods. Before you go, you might also want to turn to Emily Richards's recipe section later in this book and pick out some new dishes to try. To make your first green-light shopping excursion simpler, I've included a shopping list on page 179, which you can take with you. On it, you will find dried apricots listed – though they are yellow-light, they can be used in Emily's recipes.

I've tried to include a broad range of products in the G.I. Diet Food Guide, but of course I couldn't hope to include all the thousands of brands available in most supermarkets. Check labels when in doubt, and look for three things in particular: 1. Check the calorie content per serving and that the serving size is realistic. Some manufacturers will low-ball the serving size in order to make the calories or fat content appear lower than that of their competitors' products. 2. Check the fat content, especially of saturated fat or trans fatty acids (usually called hydrogenated), and look for a minimum ratio of 3 grams of poly- or mono-unsaturated fat to each gram of saturated fat. The total amount of fat should be less than 10 grams per serving. 3. Note the fibre content, since fibrous foods have a lower G.I. rating. Look for a minimum of 4 to 5 grams of fibre per serving. You will probably be buying more fruit and vegetables than usual, so be a little daring and try some varieties that are new to you.

STEP 4: START EATING THE GREEN-LIGHT WAY

Altering one's eating habits always requires some additional thought and preparation initially. As you begin to eat the green-light way, you will most likely have to consult the G.I. Diet Food Guide often. Before long, however, choosing the right foods will become second nature. To make starting the new plan as easy as possible, I suggest that you choose one or two standard breakfasts that you can eat every day for the first couple of weeks. This may sound boring, but you most likely do this now without thinking much about it. Perhaps you always have a bowl

Dear Rick,

I have Type 2 diabetes, hypertension and I'm over 100 pounds overweight. My husband had recently been tested for high cholesterol and needed to lose 2 stones or so. We emptied our fridge and pantry over a period of time and, armed with your excellent shopping guide, bought most of what we thought we'd need for the first week of the diet. I made up three pages of quick-reference breakfast, lunch, supper and snack ideas and taped them up in the kitchen.

We started eating right exactly eight weeks ago. My husband has lost 1½ stones and is waiting for the results of his cholesterol test. I have lost 1 stone and a few inches around my waist. But the most remarkable thing is that my sugar levels have normalized. . . . My doctor says if things continue this way, I may be able to go off insulin completely. During my checkup last week we discovered that my blood pressure was normal for the first time in years.

This is the first time that I have not felt hungry while trying to lose weight. There have been MANY challenges but your hints, especially about eating out, have made it so much easier. I keep apples, yoghurt and almonds at my two places of work and a Balance Bar and glucose tablets in my purse in case I miss a snack between jobs or if I get too busy.

I have turned at least ten people on to your marvellous book and all of them are losing weight and feeling great. Thank you for making it relatively easy for a lot of desperate people to quietly try something and succeed.

Yours sincerely,
Margie

of cornflakes with fruit, or a toasted bagel with cream cheese. Decide what you are now going to have and give yourself enough time each morning to prepare and eat it. I myself look forward to starting each day with a bowl of porridge. I vary its flavour by adding different types of fruit yoghurt or sliced fruit or berries. You'll find more breakfast ideas on pages 100 to 109.

While your dinner preparation routine is unlikely to change, lunches and snacks, because they are often eaten away from home, will require some extra forethought. As I said earlier, you can eat the green-light way at restaurants, but the best option is to brown bag it. Make any of the soups in the recipe section of this book ahead of time and store them in lunch-size quantities in the freezer. You could also prepare one of Emily's salads the night before. Another suggestion would be to make extra when you are preparing dinner and have the leftovers for lunch the next day.

Be sure to plan out your snacks as well. Keep adequate supplies of ready-to-eat snacks such as fruit yoghurt, cottage cheese, nutrition bars, fruit and nuts at home, at work, in your purse, in your briefcase and in the car. Bake other green-light snacks, such as Emily's Cranberry Cinnamon Bran Muffins, ahead of time and store them in the freezer. You can allow them to thaw in your lunch bag or defrost them in the microwave. A little preparation will ensure that you'll always have the right foods on hand when those inevitable hunger pangs strike and will go a long way in guaranteeing your success on this diet.

STEP 5: ADD SOME EXERCISE TO YOUR ROUTINE

Dieting has a far greater impact on weight loss than exercise does. To give you some idea of how much exercise is required to lose just one pound of weight, have a look at the table below.

	EFFORT REQUIRED TO LOSE 1LB OF FAT	
9-stone person	11-stone person	
Walking (4 mph–brisk)	53 miles/85 km	42 miles/67 km
Running (8 min/mile)	36 miles/58 km	29 miles/46 km
Cycling (12–14 mph)	96 miles/154 km	79 miles/127 km
Sex (moderate effort)	79 times	64 times

Clearly, an exercise regimen alone is not enough to reach your weight-loss goal, even if you are a sexual athlete! However, exercise is an important factor in *maintaining* your desired weight. For example, if you were to walk briskly for a half hour every day for one year, you would burn up calories equalling 1½ stones of fat. Exercise increases your metabolism – the rate at which you burn up calories – even after you've finished exercising! As well, it builds muscle mass, and the larger your muscles, the more energy (calories) they use. So start walking, bicycling, lifting weights, doing resistance exercises or playing sports. Not only will it help your weight-loss efforts, it will dramatically reduce your risk of heart disease, stroke, diabetes and osteoporosis.

These five steps will get you well on your way to achieving your weight-loss target. Don't be surprised if you lose more than one pound per week during the first few weeks as your body adjusts to the new plan. Most of that initial weight will be water, not fat – remember, 70 per cent of your body weight is water. Please don't worry if from time to time you 'fall off the wagon'. I probably live about 90 per cent within the programme and 10 per cent outside it. It's important that you don't feel as though you're living in a straitjacket. The fact is that I feel better and more energized when I stick to green-light foods, and you will too. Try to keep your lapses to a minimum – they will marginally delay your target date. Once you have reached your goal, you will be able to allow yourself more leeway in Phase II.

4 Phase II

When you're ready to begin Phase II of the G.I. Diet, hearty
congratulations are in order: you've reached your weight-loss
target! You stuck to the principles of the programme and are
looking and feeling great as a result. All you have to do now is
maintain your new weight. While this is definitely a less onerous
phase than the first, maintenance can also be a challenge. In
fact, those of you who have lost weight in the past only to
regain it soon after may find the thought of Phase II a daunting
prospect. I recently received an e-mail from a reader who lost 3
stones in just six months on the G.I. Diet. Though she had reached
her ideal BMI of twenty-two, she was terrified of moving into
Phase II in case she gained the weight back. Statistics tell us
that 95 per cent of people who lose weight on a diet tend to
put it back on. However, before you start feeling completely
demoralized, please be aware that the primary reason for
these bad odds is the diets themselves.

The truth is you can lose weight on virtually any diet. Yes,
it may be bad for your health and you may be half-starving,
but you will drop the pounds if you manage to stick to it. The
problem is that almost all diets – unlike the G.I. Diet – are
completely unsustainable. And research tells us that there
are three fundamental reasons why:

1. The diets are too complicated, written in incomprehensible
   jargon, and requiring dieters to count calories and measure
   and weigh portions.
2. The diets leave people feeling hungry and deprived all the time
   and unwilling to continue.
3. The diets make people feel unwell because the regimens are
   having a negative impact on their health. Many, if not most,
   diets are potentially damaging to one's health.

Clearly, it's pretty impossible to stick to a diet with any of the above characteristics. That's why I deliberately constructed the G.I. Diet to deal with each of those problems head on. First, the programme is simplicity itself. You don't have to figure out the number of calories in everything you eat. If you can follow a traffic light, you can follow this diet. Second, if you eat all the recommended meals and snacks, you will not go hungry or feel deprived. This is the core reason why people are able to stick to this diet. Third, this programme will not only do no harm to your health, it will actually benefit it. Because the G.I. Diet includes whole grains, fruits and vegetables, low-fat dairy products, protein and beneficial fats, it will actually improve your odds against today's major diseases, such as heart disease and stroke, diabetes, Alzheimer's and many forms of cancer. In summary then, the G.I. Diet addresses all the principal reasons why most diets don't work. And I guarantee that you will feel better on this diet than you ever have before.

This may be hard to believe, but when I reached my target weight after losing twenty-two pounds, I had to make a conscious effort to eat more in order to avoid losing more weight. My wife said I was entering 'the gaunt zone'! In Phase II, you must eat more than you did during the weight-loss portion of the diet in order to maintain your new weight. Remember the equation: food energy ingested must equal energy expended to keep weight stable. But I do have a few words of caution. You will require considerably less calories than you did before you started the diet because first, your body has become accustomed to doing with fewer calories and has to a certain extent adapted. Your body is more efficient than it was in the bad old days. Second,

Dear Rick,

This is a fabulous diet, if you can call it a diet. I find it's simply a different way of eating – a very simple, common-sense way of eating. For years, I've been slowly putting on weight and wondering why, and then this book explained it to me. I'd become a carbohydrate addict and was constantly eating processed foods. I've always tried to eat healthily and was even vegetarian for several years, but I found that I slowly but surely kept putting on weight. Then I happened to pick up *The G.I. Diet* in a bookstore and started flipping through it. Everything in it made so much sense.

So far, I've been on this so-called diet for just over a month, and have lost over a stone. I'm 5' 11" and was at 14 stones 9lb – on the verge of being obese. Now I'm down to 13½ stones and I haven't even started to exercise. . . . My eating habits have changed significantly. I think the biggest thing this diet has given me is the ability to tell when I'm full. I used to overeat all the time because I didn't really feel full. Now I pretty much always feel full, even when it's time to eat – and it takes a heck of a lot less for me to feel full.

I'm at the point now where if I try to indulge myself by having a treat, I pretty much always find it a letdown because my tastes have changed. I firmly believe that not all diets work for all people, but this one definitely works for me!

Phil

your slimmer body needs fewer calories to function. For example, if you lost 10 per cent of your body weight, you now require 10 per cent fewer calories.

The biggest mistake most people make when coming off a diet is to assume they can go back to eating the way they did before the diet. The reality is that you will probably need only a marginal increase in food energy to balance out the energy in/energy out equation. Only you can determine how big that increase should be. Try serving yourself slightly larger portion sizes or adding foods from the yellow-light category to your meals. Continue to monitor your weight each week, and if you start to gain, cut down a bit on the yellow-light foods; if you continue to lose, eat a bit more; if your weight remains stable, you've reached that magic balance and this is how you will eat for the rest of your life. You'll know what your body needs and you won't have to weigh yourself so often. You'll experience none of those hypoglycemic lows and will no longer crave junk food. And you'll be able to cheat once in a while without gaining any pounds. You will be in control of your weight.

Here are some suggestions for how you might wish to modify your eating pattern in Phase II.

Breakfast
- Increase cereal serving size, e.g., from 50–75g (1²/₃–2¹/₂oz) porridge.
- Add a slice of 100% whole grain toast and a pat of margarine.
- Double up on the sliced almonds on cereals.
- Help yourself to an extra slice of back bacon.
- Have a glass of juice now and then.
- Add one of the forbidden fruits – a banana or pineapple – to your cereal.

Lunch

I suggest you continue to eat lunch as you did in Phase I. This is the one meal that contained some compromises in the weight-loss portion of the programme since it is a meal that most of us buy each day.

Dinner

- Add another boiled new potato (from two or three to three or four).
- Increase the rice or pasta serving by up to 50 per cent.
- Have a 180g (6oz) steak instead of your regular 120g (4oz).
- Eat a few more olives and nuts.
- Try a cob of sweet corn with a dab of non-hydrogenated margarine.
- Have a glass of red wine with dinner.

Snacks

- Have some light microwave popcorn (the maximum serving is $1/3$ of a packet).
- Indulge in a square or two of bittersweet chocolate (see below).
- Eat a banana.
- Enjoy a scoop of low-fat ice cream.

Chocolate

This rich, luscious treat is the first thing all you chocoholics will want to incorporate back into your diet. And you can. Choose chocolate with a high-cocoa content (a minimum of 70 per cent), because it delivers more chocoholic satisfaction per gram, and have only a square or two every once in a while. Because chocolate contains large quantities of saturated fat and sugar, it is quite fattening. But you can definitely get away with a couple of squares. Nibbled slowly or dissolved in the mouth, these two squares are all you'll need to enjoy the taste and get the fix you need.

Alcohol

In Phase II, a daily glass of wine, preferably red and with dinner, is not only allowed, it's encouraged! Red wine is particularly rich in flavonoids, and when it is drunk in moderation (a glass a day), it has a demonstrable benefit in reducing the risk of heart attack and stroke.

What about beer? Well, unfortunately for all us beer aficionados, beer has an exceptionally high G.I. rating due to its malt content. Still, I do enjoy an occasional pint. Real discretion is required here. If you do drink alcohol, always have it with a meal. Food slows down the absorption of alcohol, thereby minimizing its impact.

With all these new options in Phase II, the temptation may be to overdo it. Remember to continue to weigh yourself weekly when you first begin in order to find your equilibrium. Once you do, eating the right amount will become second nature. You will find that Phase II is an easy and quite natural way to live, and that many of those high-fat foods you once thought you couldn't live without are no longer desirable.

Living the G.i. Diet

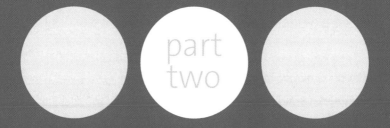

part
two

5 Coach's corner

By this point it's most likely safe to assume that you've committed yourself to the principles of the G.I. Diet and to losing weight permanently. Perhaps you've completed the five essential steps for getting started and have even begun to lose weight. Maybe you've already been on the diet for a few months and are seeing substantial results. Whatever stage you may be at, you are bound to face the inevitable dieting hurdles that test everyone's firmest resolve. Food cravings, holidays and celebrations, vacations and flagging enthusiasm are all challenges to our commitment to healthy eating. In this chapter, I will give you some tips for dealing with these dietary hazards.

FOOD CRAVINGS

What makes losing weight particularly challenging is that we tend to enjoy and desire fattening foods such as chocolate, cookies, ice cream, peanut butter, chips and so on. The most important thing to remember about cravings is that we're only human and it's natural to succumb to temptation every now and then. Don't feel guilty about it. If you 'cheat', you aren't totally blowing your diet. You're simply experiencing a temporary blip in your good eating habits. If you have a small piece of chocolate cake after dinner, or perhaps a beer with the guys while watching the game, make sure you savour the extravagance by eating or drinking *slowly*. Really enjoy it. Then get back on track in the morning with a green-light breakfast and stick to the straight and narrow for the next couple of weeks. You will continue to lose weight, and that's what it's all about.

A friend of mine, who is a cardiologist, allows himself a few 'red days' a month. These are days when he knows he has strayed from the guidelines of the G.I. Diet. To prevent red days from becoming a habit, he monitors them by marking them on his calendar. The G.I. Diet itself will help prevent lapses in two key ways. First, you will find that after you've been on the programme for a few weeks, you will have developed a built-in warning system: you won't feel good physically when you eat a red-light food because your blood sugar will spike and crash. You'll feel bloated, uncomfortable and lethargic, and you may even get a headache – a strong deterrent against straying into red-light territory. Second, because you are eating three meals and three snacks daily, you won't feel hungry between meals. If you skip any, you will probably start longing for forbidden foods – so make sure you eat all the recommended meals and snacks every day.

Despite the diet's built-in security system, there will be times when a craving gets the better of you. What should you do? Well, you could try substituting a green-light food for the red-light food you're thinking about. If you want something sweet, try having fruit; low-fat, sugar-free yoghurt; low-fat ice cream with no added sugar; any of Emily's dessert recipes; a food bar or a caffeine-free diet soft drink. If what you want is something salty and crunchy, try having a dill pickle or Emily's Dried Chickpeas (page 164). You could also make some Sage and Tomato White Bean Dip (page 164) and have it with celery sticks.

Your craving for chocolate in Phase I may be alleviated with a chocolate flavoured food bar, with light instant chocolate or with

Emily's Baked Chocolate Mousse (page 172) or Pecan Brownies (page 174). As you can see, there are many green-light versions of the foods we normally reach for when a craving strikes.

Sometimes, however, there isn't a likely substitute for the foods we miss. I have received many e-mails from readers who love peanut butter and say they cannot live without it. The thing to do here is to select the most nutritional product available – the natural kind that is made from peanuts only and has no additives such as sugar – and eat only a tablespoon of it once in a while. It's better to consume the good fats that are in peanuts than the red-light fillers that are found in other varieties of peanut butter. Don't be fooled into thinking the 'lite' versions are better for you. The amount of peanuts in these products has been reduced and sugar and starch fillers have been added. Remember that the more red-light foods you consume, the more you will slow your progress in achieving your target BMI.

HOLIDAYS AND CELEBRATIONS

We all know how much determination and gumption it takes to commit ourselves to a new weight-loss plan and how much drive it takes to clear one's cupboards, go shopping and embark on an unfamiliar way of eating. That's why once we have managed to do all this, the last thing we want is for a holiday to come along and throw a wrench into our progress. Christmas, Easter, Passover and so on all have one thing in common: an abundance of food. Holidays are generally centred around traditional feasts and dishes. But even so, you don't have to throw the G.I. guidelines out the window. You can stay in the green and still have a fun and festive holiday.

If you host the event yourself, you will be able to decide what type of food is served. Think of what you would normally eat during the holiday and look for green-light alternatives. For example, if you usually have a roast turkey with bread-based stuffing for Christmas, have a roast turkey with wild or basmati rice stuffing instead. If you always make cranberry sauce with sugar, prepare it with a sweetener. My wife, Ruth, and I always add slivered almonds and chunks of orange to our cranberry sauce – delicious! There is no shortage of green-light vegetables to serve as side dishes, and dessert can be elegant poached pears or a pavlova with berries. You can put on a completely green-light feast without your guests even realizing.

If you celebrate the holiday at someone else's home, you will obviously have less control over the menu. You could help out the busy host by offering to bring a vegetable side dish or the dessert – a green-light one, of course. Once seated at the holiday table, survey the dishes and try to compose your plate as you would at home: vegetables on half the plate, rice or pasta on one quarter and a source of protein on the other. Pass on the rolls and mashed potatoes – have extra vegetables instead. If you wish, you can allow yourself a concession by having a small serving of dessert. If you aren't particularly big on sweets, you might prefer to have a glass of wine instead. Try not to indulge in both.

Cocktail parties can also be fun, green-light occasions. Instead of alcohol, you can have a glass of mineral water with a twist of lemon or a diet caffeine-free soft drink. If you really would like an alcoholic beverage, have only one and try to choose the least red-light option. Red wine is your best bet, or a white wine spritzer made half with wine and half with sparkling water. Be sure to consume any alcohol with food to slow down the rate at which you metabolize it. Beer has a very high G.I. rating, so that's a real concession. Have it if you really want it, but make sure it's only one. Other drinks are also high G.I. and high calorie.

If you host the cocktail party yourself, you can make all the appetizers green-light. Have a cooked, sliced turkey as a centrepiece and offer lean sliced deli ham with a selection of mustards. Serve a variety of raw vegetables with a choice of low-fat dips and salsa. Hummus with wedges of whole wheat pita, smoked salmon or caviar on cucumber slices, crab salad on snow peas, chicken or beef skewers, meatballs made with extra-lean ground beef, and sashimi with soy sauce all make wonderful appetizers that everyone will enjoy. You can also provide bowls of nuts and olives, but remember to have only a few of each and don't linger nearby – it's too tempting to keep munching as you chat with your guests. Be sure to also serve a platter piled decoratively with a wide variety of green-light fruits.

If you are attending someone else's cocktail party, have a green-light meal before you go so you won't be tempted to eat too much. Then choose the low-G.I. appetizers and enjoy your time with friends and family.

HOLIDAYS AND DINING OUT

Going away on holiday usually means having to eat all your meals at restaurants – unless you spend a week at a cottage or a beach house where you can do the cooking yourself. It's not terribly difficult, though, to put the G.I. guidelines into practice when dining out. First of all, you must ask the server not to leave the habitual basket of bread or rolls on your table. If it's not there, you won't be tempted.

Order a green salad to start and choose a low-fat dressing to be served on the side so that you can control the amount you use. Salads have a very low-G.I. rating (if made with low-G.I. ingredients) and will help to fill you up before the main course arrives, so you won't be tempted to overeat. Then order an entree that includes a low-fat source of protein. Since boiled new potatoes are rarely available and you may not be sure what sort of rice is being used, ask for double the amount of vegetables instead. I've made this request in hundreds of restaurants and have never been refused. On page 183, I have included a detachable summary of dining out tips that you can keep in your wallet or purse.

When the server brings you the healthy, green-light meal you ordered, be sure to eat it slowly. There is a distinct connection between the speed at which we eat our food and feeling full or satiated. The stomach can take twenty to thirty minutes to let the brain know when it feels full. So you may be shovelling in more food than you require before your brain says stop. The other day, a friend of mine, who is a physician, noted that one of the common traits among his overweight physician colleagues was that they tended to bolt down their food. He thought that the habit probably stemmed from the days when they were busy residents and had to eat as quickly as they could in the hectic hospital environment. The famous Dr Samuel Johnson in the eighteenth century advised chewing food thirty-two times before swallowing it! That's probably going overboard, but at least put your fork down between mouthfuls. If you savour your food by eating more slowly, you will leave the table feeling far more satisfied – you'll be amazed at the difference it makes.

Just because you are on holiday doesn't mean you shouldn't continue to eat three meals and three snacks daily. In your suitcase, pack some green-light snacks to take with you, such as food bars, nuts and any other non-perishables. Once there, you can buy non-fat, sugar-free yoghurt, fruit and low-fat cottage cheese to snack on. Avoid the Continental breakfasts offered in some hotels. They are generally made up of red-light foods and offer little in the way of nutrition. One option for breakfast is to buy your own fruit, green-light cereals and milk at a supermarket and have breakfast in your hotel room.

If you are driving to your destination or are going on a road trip, your only option along the highway may be fast food. If you can, pack some green-light meals and snacks to take with you, so you won't have to stop to eat. Otherwise, I have provided some tips for eating at fast food outlets on pages 39–40.

STAYING MOTIVATED

Losing weight takes time and patience. If it took you five years to gain twenty pounds, how can you expect to lose them in the space of a month? Most people tend to lose the first few pounds very quickly. But as your body adjusts to the new way of eating, you may have a week where you won't lose, while other weeks you may lose two or three pounds. Remember that it's the average that counts, and you should target an average of *one pound per week*. How do you stay motivated for the time it takes to reach your BMI target? In my first book, *The G.I. Diet*, I listed a number of tips that are worth repeating here.

1. Maintain your weekly progress log. Success is a powerful motivator.
2. Set up a reward system. Buy yourself a small gift when you achieve a predetermined weight goal – perhaps a gift for every three pounds lost.
3. Identify family members or friends who will be your cheerleaders. Make them active participants in your plan. Or, find a friend who will join the plan for mutual support.
4. Avoid acquaintances and haunts that may encourage your old behaviours. You know who I mean!
5. Try adding what my wife, Ruth, calls a special 'spa' day to your week – a day when you are especially good with your programme. This will give you some extra credit in your weight-loss account to draw on when the inevitable relapse occurs.
6. Check out **www.gidiet.co.uk** to read about other dieters' experiences, to share your own and to keep updated on new developments.

YOUR HEALTH

If your enthusiasm starts to flag, try to remember what you were thinking and feeling the day you decided to start the G.I. Diet. You were probably feeling fed up and wishing you were slim. You were probably concerned about your health, too. And you had good reason to be. The fatter you are, the more likely it is that you will suffer a heart attack or stroke, develop diabetes and raise your risk for many cancers.

The two key factors linking heart disease and stroke to diet are cholesterol and hypertension (high blood pressure). High cholesterol is the key ingredient in the plaque that can build up in your arteries, eventually cutting off the supply of blood to your heart (causing heart attack) or your brain (leading to stroke). Hypertension puts more stress on the arterial system, causing it to age and deteriorate more rapidly, ultimately leading to arterial damage, blood clots, and heart attack or stroke. Excess weight has a major bearing on high blood pressure. A Canadian study in 1997 found that obese adults, aged eighteen to fifty-five, had a five- to thirteen-times greater risk of hypertension.

Diabetes is the kissing cousin of heart disease in that more people die from heart complications arising from diabetes than from diabetes alone. And diabetes rates are skyrocketing: they are expected to double in the next ten years. The principal causes of the most common form of diabetes, Type 2, are obesity and lack of exercise, and the current epidemic is strongly correlated to the obesity trend.

Being overweight has also been linked to cancer. A recent global report by the American Institute for Cancer Research concluded that 30 to 40 per cent of cancers are directly linked to dietary choices. Its key recommendation is that individuals should choose a predominantly plant-based diet that includes a variety of vegetables, fruits and whole grains – basically what the G.I. Diet recommends. So please do stick with it. Your weight has tremendous bearing on your health. What's worth more to you, a hamburger and fries or a long, healthy life to be shared with loved ones? I think the choice is obvious.

Dear Rick,

I am writing this testimonial to your diet on behalf of my mother who is 79 years young and very grateful for your book. She was diagnosed with diabetes last spring . . . and was a candidate for a heart attack. She was very worried. Her doctor gave her six months to do something about it through diet and exercise before putting her on insulin. He prescribed your book and wished her luck.

She was so afraid of having to take insulin every day that she was really motivated to follow your recommendations. She did so faithfully and has lost 1 stone 9lb! More importantly, her blood sugar has gone down to 4. . . . She is completely convinced of the value of your programme and tells everyone about it. . . . From my perspective, as a daughter who cherishes her mum, I can't tell you how happy it makes me when my mother shows me yet another garment that needs to be made smaller because of her success. Her pride and sense of accomplishment only enhance an already special lady, and I thank you for it.

Monique

6 The G.i. Family

As I mentioned in the previous chapter, one way of staying motivated on the G.I. Diet is to get a family member on board. If both of you are trying to lose weight together, you can support each other and have fun while doing so. More often than not, the letters I receive tell me about the results both husband and wife are seeing now that they're on the programme together. But not everyone has someone in his or her family who wants or needs to lose weight. Does that mean they have to prepare separate meals for themselves? The answer is absolutely not.

The G.I. Diet is suitable for the whole family because it's really not a diet at all – it's simply a very healthy way of eating, based on real, everyday foods. Phase II is the way we should eat throughout our entire lives. A friend of mine who went on the G.I. Diet began serving herself and her husband green-light meals for dinner every night without telling him they were based on the G.I. guidelines. He never even realized he was eating according to the recommendations of a diet plan!

Phase II is also an ideal way for children to eat – and not just those who need to lose weight. We all know that the number of overweight and obese Britons has risen dramatically in the last several years due to poor eating habits and lack of physical activity. Unfortunately, being overweight has become all too common among children. Childhood overweight and obesity has doubled in a decade. That's why it's so important to start introducing good eating habits to your children early on – it will serve them well in the future. Don't you wish you had never been introduced to junk food? If you had never had it, you wouldn't miss it now. If children don't get used to sugary soft drinks and candy, they won't develop cravings for these things later on.

We have found in our home that kids adapt easily to the G.I. way of eating. They like green-light foods and don't feel deprived. Of course, this doesn't mean that your children shouldn't be allowed to enjoy their Halloween treats or birthday cake and ice cream. It's just that these things should be saved for special occasions. On the average day, children should eat a nutritious breakfast (not sugary cereals or Pop Tarts!), lunch and dinner and snacks based on the G.I. guidelines. Fresh fruit, vegetables, fish, chicken, yoghurt, whole wheat bread, porridge, and apple bran muffins are all kid-friendly food. Just remember that growing children need sufficient fat in their diet – the good kind of fat found in fish, nuts and vegetable oils.

From the beginning, we made a point of serving our children healthy meals and snacks. We didn't keep soft drinks and other junk food in the house, but we didn't try to police our children either. Halloween always meant a period of 'sugar shock,' and birthday cakes were always decorated with Smarties. But the rest of the party food we served was nutritious – sandwiches made with whole wheat bread, vegetables with dips, and fruit – and loot bags contained little candy if any. Our son David loved having porridge and yoghurt for breakfast, although the consistency of it was always a matter of much negotiation: not too lumpy, not too smooth. We always tried to sit down for dinner as a family and catch up on what was happening with everyone. We never used dessert to bribe them to eat, and we usually served fruit for that course.

Our boys participated in making nutritious snacks. We have photos of the early muffin-makers replete with long aprons and large wooden spoons. They also enjoyed having raw vegetables for snacks if they were accompanied by interesting, low-fat dips. Now as adults, our sons continue to eat healthy diets and do not suffer from cravings for sweets or fast food. They love seafood, eat a wide variety of vegetables and like to introduce their parents to new green-light foods. We first tried edamame pods at my eldest son's home.

So if you haven't yet done so, try serving all your family members green- and yellow-light meals. Don't tell them that they are following the G.I. Diet, just say that you'd like everyone to try eating a healthier way. The early experiences children have with food have tremendous impact on the way they will eat as adults – a trend that my wife, Ruth, happens to know a great deal about. She is a professor at the University of Toronto and specializes in childhood trauma and its effects on behaviour later in life. In the next chapter, she will talk about the role food plays in our upbringing and how we learn to comfort ourselves with it.

Dear Rick,
As a teenager I know that dieting is a big thing for a lot of us. So many of my friends are always trying different diets to lose weight and usually end up going hungry. Because I've witnessed this happen so many times, the idea of dieting completely turned me off – until I found your diet. Considering this was the first diet I'd really ever done, I'm surprised that it actually worked. I've been so amazed with the results, I don't want to give away my secret to my friends! I've managed to lose 1 stone 10lb in a healthy, natural way – even my doctor is pleased with what I have done.

I just wanted to commend you on this wonderful diet.
Trust me, I'm never hungry.
Erika

7 Food as Comfort

As soon as we are born, food and comfort become permanently intertwined. From the moment we are held secure by our mothers and fed snug in their arms, food will always be connected with being held, being safe and being comforted. And these connections stay with us for the rest of our lives.

As we grow, food continues to play a vital role in our relationship with our parents, especially our mothers, since they traditionally have been the preparers of food. Their success or failure as mothers is often judged by the plumpness of their children. Thin babies are considered 'malnourished' and, even worse, 'neglected' and 'uncared for' by a not-good-enough mother. A plump baby with lots of cheek to pinch is perceived as a sign of successful mothering.

As we grew, our milestones were marked by celebrations and parties all based around food. Even when we were ill, Mom could be trusted to make a special effort to feed us foods that would encourage our appetites. When we ourselves became parents, we used food, candy or visits to fast-food restaurants to bribe our children to be good on outings and as rewards for toilet training. Our parents became eager-to-please grandparents who 'spoiled' their grandchildren with an apparent bottomless pit of food goodies.

Food permeates all aspects of our social life. It plays a role far beyond nourishing us and ensuring our continued survival. Food is a way for us to show trust, friendship and love. We celebrate holidays, such as Christmas, Passover and Easter, with food. From christenings and circumcisions to funerals and wakes, food is the one constant companion throughout our lives. In some cultures, the 'breaking of bread' together symbolizes trust, and to refuse food when offered would be perceived as an insult. As we venture forth into the world, food continues to take a central place in our social activities, such as dating and 'doing lunch' for business or pleasure. And what would a football game be without beer and pizza?

Our relationship with food, however, isn't always wonderful. Food can also be used as a weapon. Children use it as a way of rebelling against their family. Most of you can probably remember the endless battle of wills to get children to eat, often ending with food being choked down or spit up. Our youngest son went through an 'only bananas and yoghurt' phase that seemed to go on for an age but likely lasted only a week – we all survived without serious consequence. And the games we played to persuade them to eat! I can remember cutting toast into strips, dipping them into the required food at hand and flying them with aircraft sounds into our son's waiting airplane hangar (mouth). The associations we make between food and the people we love are a critical part of our developmental history.

Food can also be used to induce guilt. While the popular media make jokes about the Jewish/Greek/Italian mother who forcefeeds her children in a display of love, the message 'if you love me, you will eat my food' can be a burden. Not being able to leave the table until the overflowing food on the plate is eaten or being unable to refuse a second helping without 'hurting' the feelings of Mother can establish habits of overeating as well as conflicting feelings around food for a lifetime. Rick, for example, was taught to always eat everything on his plate and to this day finds it hard not to clean it up along with everything on the table. As a result, I have learned not to put out an excess of food – just the right amount.

Like Rick, we bring to our eating habits our unique history of early experiences and associations with food. When I'm ill, I like chicken soup with rice or tomato soup with macaroni because that's what my much-loved grandmother would feed me as a child. The soup thus comforts my stomach and my psyche, unconsciously reviving the good feelings I felt in the cared-for presence of my grandmother. This kind of connection between food and psychological nurturing is common and not something we do consciously. I don't think about my grandmother every time I eat chicken soup, but I sure feel better.

We also bring other kinds of eating habits with us. As children, many of us would come home from school and head straight to the kitchen for a snack. Now as adults, we may still head for the kitchen as soon as we come home – not just to make dinner but to have a snack. Given the hectic pace of our lives – working full time as well as somehow fitting in ferrying our children to and from child care, shopping, going to dentist appointments and so on – the ritual of walking in the door and reaching for food may be the only time during the entire day when we do something just for ourselves! Due to my British heritage, I like to come home and have a cup of tea with my afternoon green-light snack before starting the 'evening shift'. It's important to me that I always sit down and have this snack even if it's only for five minutes (it's five minutes for *me*).

Now, while we all use food as comfort or a reward to a greater or lesser extent, for some of us it can become a too-important comforter in our lives. This can put us at serious risk for overeating, weight gain and obesity. Of course there are other ways to soothe ourselves by putting things in our mouth – smoking, drinking and doing drugs being other key self-soothing behaviours. Many of these behaviours can become habits. Just as we can get into the habit of smoking, we can get into the habit of sitting down to watch television with food in hand – and as we all know, breaking a habit is very hard to do.

If you are in the habit of frequent snack eating, giving up those comfort foods is going to be a challenge, particularly since comfort foods are often junk foods, such as chips, cookies and candies, which have a high G.I. rating and therefore provide a quick sugar rush that feels good briefly. These foods do nothing to really fill you up either psychologically or physiologically and generally only leave you craving more. And so the vicious cycle continues, leaving you feeling even unhappier because of the weight gain that results.

This doesn't mean you can't snack – far from it. The G.I. Diet recommends having three snacks a day in addition to your regular three meals. It's just that your snacks are going to be different. Choose fruit, a whole range of low-fat dairy products, and home-made muesli and muffins, just to name a few options. Until you get into the habit of eating this way, these snacks may not provide the sugar rush 'comfort' and mouth-feel you rely on to feel good. So it may be helpful to start thinking about alternative ways to comfort yourself when alone in the evening after a hard day at work.

Take some time to think about how and when you eat. Do you eat on the run, standing up, taking little or no real pleasure in your eating? Are meals enjoyable social times or times of high stress and tension? Do you walk in the door after work and start eating continuously until bedtime, and are you aware you are doing this? When you really think about it, are you eating for reasons other than to alleviate hunger? Do you eat to relieve boredom, stress, anxiety or loneliness?

If this sounds like you, then you need to stop and think: are there things you can change so that mealtimes are pleasurable and tension free? Take some time to plan your meals (consider weekly meal plans) and make time for shopping and preparation. Next try to ensure that you always sit down at a table at a fairly regular time to eat your meals. Don't eat standing up or while doing other chores or tasks. Relax and enjoy your food, eating slowly. Once you have thought about ways to make meals comforting and enjoyable, you can start thinking about how you can substitute pleasurable activities for some of your snacking habits. To do this, I'd like you to draw up a list of all the activities you enjoy doing, including hobbies and pleasurable distractions. I've included an example of a list below, but yours will be unique to you.

Activities
Having a bath surrounded by candles
Listening to music
Going to a football match
Doing yoga
Going to see a movie

Hiking in the outdoors
Woodworking
Calling a friend
Fishing
Looking at old photographs
Reading a novel
Making a scrapbook
Writing a diary

Doing some of the items on your list may feel self-indulgent and a waste of time – something we've been taught is a bad thing. It's okay, a good idea even, to do pleasurable, nice things for yourself.

So the next time you feel like reaching for a red-light snack, perhaps a bowl of popcorn while watching television, do one of the activities on your list instead. Have a warm bubble bath or call a friend to chat. I know this shift sounds hard, but take it slowly and remember that the first step to any kind of change is recognizing that something needs to change. By reading this book, you've already started that process. If you have a partner, get him or her on side – the support of friends and family is essential if this is going to really work. Make sure they understand what you are trying to do and get them to help you by including them in your activities.

Food will always play an important part in our lives as a source of nutrition, in socialization and for comfort. Eating can be pleasurable and satisfying. By slowly making healthy changes to the way you eat, you will find that food has a more balanced place in your life.

Dear Rick,

I wanted to write and thank you for your book. I have been overweight all my life. . . . I had peaked at 21½ stones and had come to the conclusion that I was a food addict and that trying to lose weight was hopeless, having tried every other plan out there – or so I thought!

Thank God a very dear friend of mine found your book. Seven weeks later I weigh 19½ stones and have never felt so good. Your plan has turned off my inner demon's voice! I no longer crave sweet things . . . I haven't had ANY chocolate in seven weeks (the longest I have been without it since birth, I swear!) and I am finding the plan easy to stick to and easy to manage. Now thanks to you I KNOW I am going to get down to a healthy body weight for the first time in my life. I am 37 years old and I feel like my life is just starting. Thank you, thank you, thank you!!

Sarah

8 Frequently asked questions

Q. Can I really eat as much of the green-light foods as I want?
A. Yes you can, except where I recommend a specific serving or portion size. Serving sizes are important for green-light foods that have a higher G.I. rating or calorie content than others, such as pasta, rice, bread, nuts and meat. Let common sense be your guide and keep everything in moderation. I wouldn't recommend eating twenty oranges a day, for example, or ten green-light muffins. That's going a bit overboard.

Q. Is there any flexibility in this diet?
A. Yes, but only you can determine which rules you can break and still lose weight. Many readers tell me they can't live without certain red-light foods such as regular coffee or peanut butter. If there's a product that is that important to you, go ahead and have it, but strictly limit the quantity you consume. Have only one cup of coffee or one tablespoon of peanut butter a day. One reader told me she was on the 'Vegas' version of the G.I. Diet, meaning she had a glass of red wine every day on Phase I. She still lost thirty pounds and is wearing the same dress size she wore back in university. Although you would lose weight faster if you followed all the guidelines of the G.I. Diet, it really is okay to live only 90 per cent on the programme.

Q. I thought aspartame and some other sweeteners were bad for your health, so why are you recommending them?
A. A great deal of misinformation has been spread about sweeteners – driven mainly by the sugar lobby in the United States. All the major government and health agencies worldwide have approved the use of sweeteners and sugar substitutes and not a single peer-reviewed (scholarly) study

has identified any health risks. For those who are still concerned about the safety of artificial sweeteners, there is a comprehensive rundown on sugar substitutes in the U.S. Food and Drug Administration Consumer Magazine (see www.fda.gov).

If you're sensitive to aspartame, check out the alternatives such as Splenda (sucralose) or Hermesetas Gold (saccharine, cyclemate).

Q. Is the herbal sweetener stevia a green-light product?
A. Stevia is a South American herb that can be found in health stores. Although its popularity is growing, no long-term studies on its safety have been carried out – so I can't wholeheartedly recommend it. But it appears to be an acceptable alternative if used in moderation.

Q. I understand that peanut butter has a low G.I. If so, why is it red-light? Are the 'lite' versions more acceptable?
A. It's true that peanut butter has a low G.I. rating, but it is extremely high in fat and is calorie dense. Unfortunately, the 'lite' varieties are even worse because the amount of peanuts has been reduced and sugar and starch fillers have been added to make up the shortfall. If you are going to 'cheat' with an occasional tablespoon of peanut butter, make sure it's the natural kind that contains 100 per cent peanuts and no added sugar.

Q. Beans are listed as green-light, yet commercially tinned black bean soup is red-light. Why?

A. Beans are a classic green-light food, low in fat and high in protein and fibre. Commercially tinned bean soups, however, are highly processed and therefore high-G.I. They are cooked at extremely high temperatures to prevent spoilage. This process breaks down both the outer protective skin of the beans and the starch granules inside – something that would normally be done by your digestive system. Because of this, tinned black bean, split pea and green pea soups are all high-G.I. Try Emily's homemade bean soups instead, which are green-light and easy to make.

Q. Dried apricots and cranberries are listed as yellow-light yet they are used in some green-light recipes. Don't they raise the G.I. level of the recipes?

A. Dried fruits actually have a low-G.I. They are for the most part, however, high in calories, which is why most are listed in the red-light column. Dried apricots and cranberries have a lower calorie content, and the amount used in the recipes is so modest, they only marginally raise the calorie content, not enough to worry about.

Q. I know you should avoid drinking alcohol in Phase I, but can you use wine in recipes?

A. Absolutely! You can cook with wine even in Phase I. Adding 240ml (8fl oz) to a sauce that is going to serve four people means that each person will only be getting 60ml (2fl oz) – much less than a glass of wine. Also, most of the alcohol tends to evaporate in the cooking process.

Dear Rick,

Thank you for your continued work with the G.I. programme. I started in May, went great guns for a while and hit a plateau. Your book has changed the way I think about food and my plateau has started to crumble again and the pounds are coming off – slowly, just the way they should. I have lost 1 stone and I look and feel so much better. I still have a long way to go. My goal is another 1½ stones over the next two years.

My heart, my body and my soul thank you for your motivation and support.

Take care,

Glennda

Q. Are low-calorie foods such as rice cakes or sugar-free Jell-O green-light foods?

A. I'm afraid not. Although they don't have a lot of calories, they are digested quickly, leaving you looking for more food to keep your digestive system busy. Try to stick to green-light snacks, which are far more nutritious and satisfying.

Q. I read that many high-fat foods such as premium ice cream are in fact low-G.I. Is this true?

A. Yes it is. Fat acts as a brake on the digestive process, which means that fatty foods take longer to digest. But they are still red-light for two reasons. First, they are high in calories. Fat contains more than twice the calories per gram than protein or carbohydrates. Second, most high-fat foods contain saturated fats, which are bad for your health. Though the G.I. content of foods is a very important factor in determining whether a food is green-light or not, we must also take into account its calorie density and its impact on our health. Saturated fat is definitely a bad fat.

Q. I've been on the G.I. Diet for several weeks and have been very pleased with my progress until the last couple of weeks or so. I seem to have hit a plateau. What should I do?
A. Most people experience rapid weight loss during the first few weeks of the diet. That sets up the expectation that weight loss will continue at the same rate, but this is generally not the case. You should expect to lose an average of one pound per week. Don't be overly concerned if you hit a plateau. If you are following the G.I. Diet guidelines and are still above your recommended bmi, you will definitely reach your goal. If your plateau seems to be lasting a bit too long, think about what you have been eating lately and whether you may be straying a bit too far from the green-light column of the food guide. I received an e-mail from a reader who said he had reached a plateau and that his only indiscretion was a couple of peanut butter snacks a day. Well, the problem was that this 'indiscretion' was delivering about 3,500 calories, or a pound of fat, to his waistline every week. No wonder he had hit a plateau!

Cooking the G.i. Way

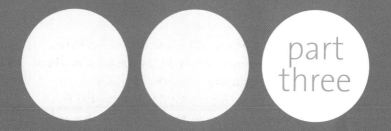

part
three

9 Introduction to G.i. Cooking

When Rick first approached me to put together a collection of recipes for his best-selling diet, I was delighted. I've always been interested in healthy cooking (I have a degree in nutrition) and have developed countless low-fat recipes for various publications over the years. Rick told me that not only would the recipes for this book have to be low in saturated fat, but they'd also have to be high fibre, low in sugar, have a low G.I. rating – and oh, taste great, too. I told him to sign me up right away! I love to create new recipes because it allows me to express my passion for cooking while 'playing' in the kitchen. And I would be helping out not only all you G.I. dieters, but also some of my own family members who have been diagnosed with diabetes, high cholesterol, high blood pressure and heart disease.

When you first begin the G.I. Diet, you may feel as though there are a lot of limitations on what you can eat. But focus on what's listed in the green-light column of the food guide, and you will see that there really is a wide-ranging variety of appealing foods. You can eat very well on the G.I. Diet and never have to sacrifice flavour. Not only are green-light foods good for you, but I also happen to think that they are some of the best tasting. Extra-virgin olive oil, for example, is a monounsaturated, or 'best', fat and adds a wonderful flavour to many dishes.

Good taste is always my primary consideration when developing new recipes. I start with my own personal experiences with food – what I enjoy cooking and what my family and friends take pleasure in eating. I like to use plenty of fresh herbs, delicious spices and ethnic flavours to come up with interesting and fun meals. In this collection, you will find some old family favourites, such as Veal Parmesan and Beef Fajitas, that I have modified to make green-light. By using less oil, avoiding white flour and sugar and using strong cheeses for flavour enhancement only, you too can turn your own much-loved recipes into green-light dishes. Ruth and Rick have shared a few of their standbys, and thanks to your e-mails, there are some readers' recipes here, too.

Cooking the G.I. way generally means cooking from scratch and avoiding heavily processed foods. But that doesn't mean you have to spend a lot of time in the kitchen. Most of the recipes in this book can be made in less than thirty minutes. I've included some breakfast recipes, such as Yoghurt Smoothies and Muesli, for those mornings when you are on the run, as well as some recipes that are more suited for relaxing weekends, like Light 'n' Fluffy Pancakes and Back Bacon Omelette. Any of the salad and soup recipes will form the basis of a satisfying lunch, and there are plenty of meatless, fish and seafood, poultry and meat dishes to choose from for dinner. And because this isn't a deprivation diet, I've also included some recipes for desserts and snacks that I'm sure you will enjoy. I've tried almost all of them out on my family, friends and cooking classes, and everyone has been amazed to discover that they are low fat and low G.I. – they taste that good. I hope that many of these green- and yellow-light dishes will become favourites among your own family and friends. In the following sections, I have included some tips on ingredients, equipment, measuring and side dishes, and have given you a week-long menu plan to help you get started.

INGREDIENTS

You will notice that not all of the ingredients that I have used in the recipes are strictly green-light. I've added wine for depth of flavour, as well as small amounts of sauces that contain sugar, and dried fruit. This doesn't mean that the recipe is yellow- or red-light. The quantities are so minor that they will have little to no effect on your blood sugar level. Don't feel you have to omit them to stay in the green.

To replace sugar in recipes, I've had great success with Splenda and have found the flavour quite good. Look for the granular type that comes in boxes because it is the easiest to use – you can measure out the amount just like sugar.

EQUIPMENT

Non-stick frying pans
When cooking low-fat dishes, it's useful to have a few non-stick skillets on hand in various sizes. You only need a minimal amount of oil when using them and food slides right off the pan. Remember that the recommended cooking heat for non-stick surfaces is no higher than medium-high and that you should use non-abrasive utensils and brushes only. Wash your skillet with hot soapy water and a nylon brush – do not put it in the dishwasher, which will damage the non-stick coating. If you need to stick your skillet in the oven and it has a plastic or wood handle, be sure to wrap the handle well with aluminum foil first.

Dear Rick,

I just wanted you to know that I saw your interview with Vicki Gabereau earlier today. My daughter and I started the G.I. Diet a couple months ago, and I have lost over a stone and my daughter has lost almost the same . . . We love the food! Old habits are certainly hard to change, but having food prepared ahead of time sure makes a difference when one is short on time. If I make batches of soup, chili and granola bars, I can be very good. However, if I haven't made some things ahead of time, it is soooo easy to fall back on old familiar (but harmful) eating patterns!

The big discovery for me was to find out how awful I feel when I go off your plan and start grabbing sweets or some such thing for a day! Y-U-C-K. I can't believe that I used to feel like that all the time before your book! I never would have thought that yoghurt would become such a good friend.

Thanks again,

Bernice

And if there is wear and tear on your pans, consider buying new ones for better performance.

Grill pan/Indoor grill

The tips I gave above for caring for your non-stick pans also apply to grill pans and indoor grills. When using them, you only need a light brush or spray of oil. A grill pan keeps the food you are cooking out of the fat and gives that grilled look when you don't have an outdoor barbecue.

Pots and pans

Ever wondered what the difference is between a pot and a pan?
Well, a pot usually has two handles and a pan has only one. They
can pretty much be used interchangeably. A Dutch oven is just a
large pan or pot that has a lid – most people have one without
even realizing it!

SIDE DISHES

Almost all of the dinner recipes I have included in this book
should be accompanied by side dishes. A quarter of your plate
should be filled with a starchy carbohydrate such as pasta, rice
or boiled new potatoes. Since overcooking tends to raise the
G.I. level of food, boil pasta until it is just 'al dente', or still firm
when bitten, and take rice off the heat before it starts to clump
together. Small new potatoes will only take about ten minutes
to boil or steam.

Half your plate should be filled with green-light vegetables and
salad. Again, do not overcook the veggies; they should be tender-
crisp. Most people I know are not avid fans of mushy, flavourless
vegetables anyway. Here are some hints for preparing your
side vegetables.

Vegetable Steaming Chart

VEGETABLE	PREPARATION
Asparagus	trim ends
Broccoli	cut into florets
Brussels sprouts	trim and halve
Carrots	cut into ½-inch chunks
Cauliflower	cut into florets
Courgettes	cut into chunks
Frozen green peas	do not thaw
Frozen mixed vegetables	do not thaw in bags
Green beans	trim tips
New potatoes	scrub and prick with fork
Sugar snap/mangetout peas	trim tips
Yellow beans	trim tips

You can cook these vegetables in any of the following ways.
To boil vegetables: In a saucepan of boiling water, cook the vegetables for about 7 minutes or until they are just tender.
To steam vegetables: In a saucepan, boil 3 cm (1in) of water. Place a steamer basket filled with the vegetables in the saucepan. Cover and steam for 5 to 7 minutes or until the vegetables are just tender.
To microwave vegetables: Place the vegetables in a large plate or bowl. Add 60ml (2fl oz) of water. Cover with clingfilm and microwave on High for about 5 minutes or until the vegetables are just tender. To dress them up and add some zing to vegetables, drizzle them with lemon juice and add salt and pepper.

SALADS

The following recipe makes a good basic salad and vinaigrette that you can endlessly vary by using different vegetables, vinegars and herbs.

Basic Salad

60g (2oz)	lettuce (such as cos, rocket, watercress, iceberg or mixed leaf)
1	small carrot, shredded
Half	a pepper (red, yellow or green)
1	plum tomato, cut in wedges
¼	sliced cucumber
2	slices of red onion (optional)

In a bowl, toss together the lettuce, carrot, pepper, tomato, cucumber and onion. Makes 1 serving.

Basic Vinaigrette

1 tbsp	vinegar (such as white or red wine, balsamic, rice or cider) or lemon juice
1 tsp	extra virgin olive or rapeseed oil
½ tsp	Dijon mustard
Pinch	each of salt and pepper
Pinch	of dried or fresh herb of choice (such as thyme, oregano, basil, Italian seasoning, marjoram, mint)

In a small bowl, whisk together the vinegar, oil, mustard, salt, pepper and herb. Pour the dressing over the salad and toss. Makes enough for 1 serving.

A SAMPLE ONE-WEEK
GREEN-LIGHT MENU PLAN

DAY 1:

Breakfast Muesli (page 115)

Snack   Cranberry Cinnamon Bran Muffin (page 168)

Lunch   Mushroom Barley and Beef Soup (page 114)

           Open-face turkey sandwich with Sage and
           Tomato White Bean Dip (page 164)

           Carrot and celery sticks

Snack   Orange and fat- and sugar-free fruit-flavoured yoghurt

Dinner   Hunter-Style Chicken (page 148)

           Long-grain rice and asparagus

Snack   Basmati Rice Pudding (page 171)

DAY 2:

Breakfast Homey Oatmeal (page 104)

           Grapefruit sections with low-fat cottage cheese

Snack   Cranberry Cinnamon Bran Muffin (page 168)

Lunch   Tuscan White Bean Soup (page 110)

           Barbecue Chicken Salad (page 126)

           Wholemeal pita half

Snack   Apple and 1% cottage cheese

Dinner   Almond Haddock Fillets (page 138)

           Baby carrots and long-grain rice

           Courgette Salad (page 120)

Snack   Apple Pie Cookie (page 173)

DAY 3:

Breakfast Back Bacon Omelette (page 108)

           Slice of 100% stone-ground wholemeal toast

           Tomato wedges

Snack   Wholemeal Scone (page 167)

Lunch   Lemon Dill Lentil Salad (page 124)

Open-face ham sandwich with Roasted Red
Pepper Hummus (page 165)
Pickle
Snack   Apple Pie Cookie (page 173) and glass of skimmed milk
Dinner   Asian Greens and Tofu Stir-fry (page 134)
Basmati rice
Tossed salad
Snack   Fresh Fruit Bowl (page 165)

DAY 4:
Breakfast Muesli (page 115)
Back bacon
Slice of 100% stone-ground wholemeal toast
Sliced peach
Snack   Wholemeal Scone (page 167)
Lunch   Ham and Lentil Soup (page 112)
Tangy Red and Green Coleslaw (page 119)
Wholemeal pita half
Snack   Baby carrots, broccoli and cucumber with
Roasted Red Pepper Hummus (page 165)
Dinner   Horseradish Burger (page 152)
Mediterranean Bean Salad (page 123)
Snack   Pecan Brownie (page 174) and glass of skimmed milk

DAY 5:
Breakfast Cinnamon French Toast (page 105)
Sliced ham
Orange
Snack   Almond Bran Haystack (page 173) and glass of skimmed milk
Lunch   Crab Salad in Tomato Shells (page 127)
Cottage cheese with apple sauce
Snack   Peach and fat- and sugar-free fruit-flavoured yoghurt
Dinner   Veal with Fennel and Mushrooms (page 158)
Spaghetti
Steamed baby carrots

	Tomato Zucchini Wheat Berry Salad (page 156)
Snack	Berry Crumble (page 171)

DAY 6:

Breakfast	Puffy Baked Apple Omelette (page 107)
	Back bacon
Snack	Almond Bran Haystack (page 173) and a glass of
	skimmed milk
Lunch	Pepper and Tomato Beef Salad (page 128)
Snack	Tofu pudding
Dinner	Easy Bake Lasagne (page 136)
	Tossed salad
Snack	Poached Pears (page 170) with
	sweetened Yoghurt Cheese (page 101)

DAY 7:

Breakfast	Morning Glory Poached Fruit (page 103)
	Florentine Frittata (page 108)
	Slice of 100% stone-ground wholemeal toast
Snack	Fat- and sugar-free fruit-flavoured yoghurt
Lunch	Avocado and Fresh Fruit Salad (page 122)
	Open-face chicken sandwich with Roasted Red
	Pepper Hummus (page 165)
Snack	Dried Chickpeas (page 164)
Dinner	Salmon Steaks with Light Dill Tartar Sauce (page 141)
	Green beans and new potatoes
	Creamy Cucumber Salad (page 117)
Snack	Glazed Apple Tart (page 172)

10 The Recipes

BREAKFAST

YOGHURT SMOOTHIES

You don't need an expensive appliance to make these fruit-flavoured smoothies – a simple whisk will do.

450ml (¾ pint) skimmed milk
1 carton (175g) fat-free, sugar-free
fruit-flavoured yoghurt
½ tsp sweetener

1. In a tall glass or small bowl, whisk together the milk, yoghurt and sugar substitute until smooth.

Makes 2 servings.

OPTIONS
Thicker Smoothies: Break out the blender and add 240g (8oz) sliced strawberries or raspberries.
Dessert Smoothies: Use 240g (8oz) low-fat, no-added-sugar ice cream instead of the yoghurt and blend with the milk, omitting the sweetener.

YOGHURT CHEESE

This can be used as a tasty spread for wholemeal toast in the morning, as a dip, or as a topping for a dessert. Yoghurt cheese is also a great substitute for sour cream in most recipes.

1 carton (750g) plain low-fat yoghurt

1. Empty the yoghurt into a cheesecloth-lined or clean tea-towel-lined sieve. Place it over large bowl. Cover it all with clingfilm and refrigerate for at least 4 hours or overnight. Discard any liquid and place the yoghurt cheese in an airtight container.

Makes 350g (12oz).

OPTIONS
Sweet Yoghurt Cheese: You can sweeten your yoghurt cheese by adding some sweetener to taste.
Lemony Yoghurt Cheese: Add 1 tsp grated lemon rind and 2 tsp lemon juice along with the sweetner to taste.
Quick Yoghurt Cheese Dip: Simply add 2 spring onions, chopped; 1 small clove garlic, crushed; 1 tbsp lemon juice; and 1 tbsp chopped fresh oregano (or 1 tsp dried) to the yoghurt cheese.

HELPFUL HINT: Keep the container the yoghurt came in and write down the best-before date – that's how long your yoghurt cheese is good for.

MUESLI ●

My friend Lesleigh introduced me to this delicious and healthy start to the day. Be sure to prepare it the night before so that it's ready to enjoy in the morning. Combine 75g (2½oz) of the Muesli with 60ml (2fl oz) of skimmed milk or water, and cover and refrigerate overnight. Then in the morning, combine the mixture with 1 carton (175g) of fat-free, sugar-free fruit yoghurt and enjoy it cold, or pop it in the microwave for a hot breakfast.

210g (7oz) large-flake oats	60g (2oz) unsalted sunflower seeds
90g (3oz) oat bran	2 tbsp wheat germ
90g (3oz) sliced almonds	¼ tsp cinnamon

1. In a large, resealable plastic bag, combine the oats, oat bran, almonds, sunflower seeds, wheat germ and cinnamon. Using a rolling pin, crush the mixture into coarse crumbs. Shake the bag to combine the mixture.

Makes 450g (1lb).

Storage: Keep in a resealable bag or airtight container at room temperature for up to 1 month.

WHEAT GRAIN BREAKFAST

This recipe comes from G.I. dieter Gwyneth, who has been making it for many years – especially during canoe trips. You can buy wheat grain, also known as soft or hard wheat kernels, at health or bulk food stores. Letting them sit overnight allows them to crack open, producing a delicate kernel of wheat.

240g (8oz) wheat grain	Sweetener
1litre (2pints) water	Sliced almonds
Skimmed milk	Fresh fruit (such as berries or peaches)

1. Place the wheat grain and water in a saucepan and bring to the boil. Reduce the heat and simmer for 20 minutes.

2. Pour the wheat grain and water into a large Thermos, or heatproof airtight container and seal tightly. Let it stand overnight.

3. Drain any water from the wheat grain. Serve about 90g (3oz) of them with milk, sweetener, almonds and fruit as desired.

Makes about 3 servings.

Helpful Hint: If there are any leftovers, be sure to refrigerate them.

MORNING GLORY POACHED FRUIT

If you don't have time to eat breakfast at home, make this fruit dish the night before, or a few days before, and take it with you. It also makes a wonderful mid-morning or mid-afternoon snack.

2 apples, cored and coarsely chopped
2 pears, cored and coarsely chopped
1 grapefruit
1 orange
450g (1lb) low-fat cottage cheese or Yoghurt Cheese
(see recipe on page 101)

Cinnamon Syrup:
450ml (¾ pint) water
2 cinnamon sticks, broken in half
4 slices fresh ginger
3 tbsp sweetener

1. Cinnamon Syrup: In a small saucepan, bring the water, cinnamon sticks, ginger and sweetener to the boil. Reduce the heat to simmer and add the apples and pears. Cook the fruit for about 5 minutes or until just tender. Remove the fruit with a slotted spoon to a large bowl, reserving the syrup. Let it cool.

2. Meanwhile, using a serrated knife, cut both ends off the grapefruit. Starting at one end, peel the skin and white pith off the grapefruit, leaving the fruit intact. Repeat with the orange. Using the same knife, cut the segments between the membranes of the grapefruit and orange and add, along with juices, to the bowl containing the apples and pears. Serve with cottage cheese and drizzle with some of the Cinnamon Syrup, if desired.

Makes 4 servings.

Storage: You can make this mixture up to 3 days ahead. Store it in an airtight container in the refrigerator.

HOMEY OATMEAL

This hot breakfast is guaranteed to keep you feeling satisfied all morning.
You can vary the flavour by topping it with fresh fruit such as berries or
chopped apple.

450ml (¾ pint) skimmed milk
325ml (12fl oz) water
I tsp cinnamon
½ tsp salt
150g (5oz) large-flake oats
30g (1oz) wheat germ
30g (1oz) chopped almonds
3 tbsp sweetener

1. In a large saucepan, bring the milk, water, cinnamon and salt to the
boil. Stir in the oats and wheat germ and return to the boil. Reduce the
heat to low and cook, stirring, for about 8 minutes or until the mixture
has thickened. Stir in the almonds and sweetener.

Makes 4 servings.

BUTTERMILK PANCAKES

This recipe comes from Michelle R. Though buttermilk may sound as
though it's rich and indulgent, it's actually low in fat and adds a
wonderful tang to these pancakes.

240g (8oz) wholemeal flour
1 tbsp baking powder
2 tsp sweetener
450ml (¾ pint) buttermilk

2 omega-3 eggs
2 tbsp rapeseed oil
½ tsp vanilla essence

1. In a large bowl, combine the wholemeal flour, baking powder and
sweetener. In another bowl, whisk together the buttermilk, eggs, rapeseed
oil and vanilla essence. Pour the buttermilk mixture over the flour mixture
and whisk together until smooth.

2. Heat a large non-stick frying pan over a medium heat. Ladle the batter
into the pan. Cook it for about 2 minutes or until bubbles appear on top
of the pancake. Using a spatula, flip the pancake and cook for another
minute or until golden. Repeat with the remaining batter.

Makes about 16 pancakes, enough for 4 to 6 servings.

CINNAMON FRENCH TOAST ●

Serve this family favourite with slices of ham or back bacon and extra strawberries for a complete breakfast.

1 omega-3 egg
3 egg whites
120ml (4fl oz) skimmed milk
1 tbsp sweetener
1 tsp vanilla essence
½ tsp cinnamon, ground
Pinch of salt
4 slices stone-ground wholemeal bread
1 tsp rapeseed oil
300g (10oz) sliced strawberries
120g (4oz) fat-free, sugar-free, fruit-flavoured yoghurt

1. In a shallow dish, whisk together the egg, egg whites, milk, sweetener, vanilla essence, cinnamon and salt. Dip each slice of bread into the egg mixture, making sure to coat both sides.

2. Meanwhile, brush a large non-stick frying pan with oil and place over a medium-high heat. Cook the bread for about 4 minutes, turning once, or until golden brown. Serve each slice with strawberries and yoghurt.

Makes 2 servings.

LIGHT 'N' FLUFFY PANCAKES

Pancakes make weekend mornings special. You can also enjoy them during the work week by making and freezing them ahead of time. When Tuesday or Wednesday rolls around, simply pop the frozen pancakes into your toaster or microwave and enjoy.

150g (5oz) plain flour
90g (3oz) wholemeal flour
15g (½oz) wheat bran
1 tbsp baking powder
¼ tsp salt
¼ tsp nutmeg

350ml (12fl oz) skimmed milk
3 omega-3 eggs
2 tbsp rapeseed oil
2 tbsp sweetener
1 tsp vanilla essence

1. In a large bowl, combine the plain and wholemeal flours, bran, baking powder, salt and nutmeg. In another bowl, whisk together the milk, eggs, oil, sweetener and vanilla essence. Pour the milk mixture over the flour mixture and whisk together until smooth.

2. Heat a large non-stick frying pan over medium heat. Ladle the batter into the pan. Cook the pancake for about 2 minutes or until bubbles appear on top. Using a spatula, flip the pancake and cook for another minute or until golden. Repeat with the remaining batter.

Makes about 16 pancakes, enough for 4 to 6 servings.

Storage: These pancakes can be frozen in a single layer on a baking sheet until firm. Place them in an airtight container once frozen.

BERRY CREPES

Crepes may sound difficult to make, but they are actually quite simple. Just make sure the pan is hot when you add the crepe batter. It should start to set as soon as you swirl it around the pan.

60g (2oz) wholemeal flour
1 tbsp ground flax seed or wheat germ
Pinch of salt
240ml (8fl oz) skimmed milk
3 omega-3 eggs
1 tsp vanilla essence
1 tsp rapeseed oil

275g (9oz) each fresh blueberries and raspberries
2 tbsp sweetener
1 tbsp chopped fresh mint (optional)
Pinch of cinnamon, ground
240g (8oz) Yoghurt Cheese (see page 101)

1. In a bowl, combine the flour, flax seed and salt. In another bowl, whisk together the milk, eggs and vanilla essence. Pour this over the flour mixture and whisk until smooth. Let the batter stand at room temperature for at least 15 minutes, or cover and refrigerate it for up to 2 hours.

2. Brush a small non-stick frying pan with some of the oil and heat over a medium heat. Pour in about 2tbsp of the batter, swirling the pan to cover the bottom. Cook the pancake for about 2 minutes or until firm and slightly golden. Turn and cook the other side for another 30 seconds. Put the pancake on a plate and repeat the process with the remaining batter.

3. In a large bowl, combine the blueberries, raspberries, sweetener, mint (if using) and cinnamon. Put about 60–90g (2–3oz) of the berry mixture in the centre of each crepe and roll up. Serve with the Yoghurt Cheese and remaining berries.

Makes about 10 crepes, enough for 4 servings.

Note: Sometimes the first crepe doesn't work out, so the recipe gives you a bit of extra batter to practise. If you're a pro at it, you'll have another serving of crepes.

PUFFY BAKED APPLE OMELETTE

You can replace the apple in this recipe with your favourite seasonal fruit. Try peaches or pears.

4 cooking apples, cored
2 tsp non-hydrogenated soft margarine
90ml (3fl oz) apple juice
¼ tsp nutmeg, ground
Pinch each of allspice and cloves
4 omega-3 eggs

5 egg whites
120ml (4fl oz) skimmed milk
50g (1²⁄₃oz) large-flake oats
30g (1oz) wholemeal flour
½ tsp salt

1. Cut each apple into 8 slices. Meanwhile, in a large non-stick frying pan, heat the margarine over a medium heat; add the apple slices, apple juice, nutmeg, allspice and cloves. Cook for about 15 minutes or until just tender. Place the apple slices into a 20-cm (8-inch) square baking dish and set aside.

2. In a large bowl, whisk together the eggs, milk, oats, flour and salt. Pour the mixture over the apples and bake at 180°C/Gas Mark 4 pre-heated oven for about 20 minutes, or until puffed and golden brown and a knife inserted in the centre comes out clean.

Makes 4 servings.

Speedy Option: Substitute a large can of sliced peaches or pears in water or fruit juice, drained, for the apples – no cooking required.

BACK BACON OMELETTE

The smoky flavour of bacon makes this omelette a hit. Serve this with fresh fruit and yoghurt for a hearty breakfast.

1 tsp rapeseed oil
1 omega-3 eggs
1 tbsp chopped fresh basil or ½ tsp dried
1 tbsp grated Parmesan cheese

2 egg whites
Pinch of pepper
2 slices cooked back bacon or ham, chopped
Quarter of a red or green pepper, chopped

1. In a small non-stick frying pan, heat the oil over a medium-high heat. In a bowl, using a fork, stir together the eggs, basil, cheese and pepper. Pour the mixture into the frying pan and cook for about 5 minutes, lifting the edges to allow the uncooked egg to run underneath, until almost set.

2. Add the bacon and red or green pepper over half of the omelette. Using a spatula, fold over the other half and cook for 1 minute. Slide onto a plate.

Makes 1 serving.

FILLING OPTIONS: Try other fillings for your omelette, like 100g (3½oz) chopped, cooked spinach or Swiss chard or asparagus or 30g (1oz) light-style Swiss or havarti cheese. For seafood lovers, try 100g (3½oz) shrimps or crabmeat.

FLORENTINE FRITTATA

A frittata is an easy Italian omelette that doesn't require flipping. You just pop it under the grill to finish it off. It also makes a delicious lunch served on a slice of stone-ground wholemeal toast with a side salad.

2 tsp extra-virgin olive oil
1 small onion, diced
2 cloves garlic, crushed
1 red pepper, chopped
2 tbsp chopped fresh oregano or 2 tsp dried
1 bag (300g/11oz) fresh baby spinach
½ tsp salt
2 omega-3 eggs
5 egg whites
60ml (2fl oz) skimmed milk
Pinch of pepper

1. In a large non-stick frying pan with an ovenproof handle, heat the oil over a medium-high heat and add the onion, garlic, red pepper and oregano. Cook, stirring, for 5 minutes or until golden. Add the spinach and half of the salt; cover and cook for 2 minutes or until spinach is wilted.

2. In a bowl, whisk together the eggs, skimmed milk, remaining salt and pepper. Pour the mixture into the frying pan, stirring gently to combine it with the spinach mixture. Cook, stirring gently, for about 2 minutes, lifting the edges to allow any uncooked egg to run underneath. Cook for another 3 minutes or until the top is set. Place the frying pan under the grill for about 3 minutes or until golden brown and a knife inserted in the centre comes out clean.

Makes 2 servings.

SHRIMP AND MUSHROOM OMELETTE

This omelette is a hit with my husband on weekend mornings. It would also make a special addition to any brunch table.

240g (8oz) small raw prawns, peeled and deveined
4 tsp rapeseed oil
Half a small onion, diced
2 cloves garlic, crushed
240g (8oz) sliced mushrooms
2 tsp chopped fresh thyme leaves or ½ tsp dried
¼ tsp salt
Pinch of pepper
Half a red pepper, thinly sliced
2 omega-3 eggs
5 egg whites
15g (½oz) chopped fresh flat leaf parsley

1. In a large non-stick frying pan, heat 1 tsp of the oil over a medium-high heat; cook the prawns for about 4 minutes or until they are pink. Place them in a bowl and keep warm. Return the frying pan to a medium-high heat and add 1 tsp of the oil. Cook the onion and garlic for about 2 minutes or until starting to brown. Add the mushrooms, thyme, salt and pepper; cook, stirring, for about 8 minutes or until all the liquid is evaporated and the mushrooms are golden. Stir in the red pepper and add the mixture to the cooked prawns.

2. In the same frying pan, heat the remaining oil over a medium heat. In a bowl, using a fork, stir together the eggs and parsley. Pour the eggs into the pan and cook for about 5 minutes, lifting the edges to allow any uncooked egg to run underneath, or until set.

3. Add the prawns and mushroom mixture to one half of the omelette. Using a spatula, fold over the other half and cook for 1 minute. Slide onto a plate and cut in half.

Makes 2 servings.

SOUPS

HARICOT BEAN SOUP

This recipe comes from Beth F., who went on the G.I. Diet after hearing about it on a local radio show. She and her husband are both enjoying the new way of eating and like having this thick and nourishing soup for lunch.

3 litres (5 pints) water
325g (11oz) dry haricot beans
2 carrots, chopped
1 large onion, chopped
1 celery stalk, chopped

1 bay leaf
1 tsp salt
Pinch of pepper
Tabasco sauce (optional)

1. In a large stockpot, bring 2 litres (3½ pints) of the water and the beans to the boil. Reduce the heat and simmer for about 1 hour or until the beans are almost tender. Add the remaining water, carrots, onion, celery and bay leaf and cook for about 1 hour or until the vegetables and beans are tender. Remove the bay leaf. Add the salt and pepper. Serve with Tabasco, if desired.

Makes 4 servings.

TUSCAN WHITE BEAN SOUP

I first tried this country-style soup in Tuscany and immediately fell in love with it. I serve this soup in deep Italian ceramic soup bowls and dream I'm back in Tuscany.

1 tbsp extra-virgin olive oil
1 onion, chopped
4 cloves garlic, crushed
1 carrot, chopped
1 celery stalk, chopped
4 fresh sage leaves or ½ tsp dried

1.5 litres (2½ pints) vegetable
or chicken stock (low fat, low sodium)
2 cans (2 x 410g) cannellini or white
kidney beans, drained and rinsed
320g (10½oz) shredded kale
Pinch each of salt and pepper

1. In a large stockpot, heat the oil over a medium heat. Add the onion, garlic, carrot, celery and sage and cook for 5 minutes or until softened.

2. Add the stock, beans, kale, salt and pepper, and cook, stirring occasionally, for about 20 minutes or until the kale is tender.

Makes 4 servings.

HEARTY ONION SOUP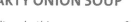

I don't make this yummy soup often enough. If you don't have French onion soup bowls, you can ladle the soup into microwave-safe bowls and melt the cheese in the microwave. Add a splash of Tabasco sauce for an added kick.

1 tbsp rapeseed oil
6 onions, thinly sliced
2 cloves garlic, crushed
½ tsp salt
2 tbsp wholemeal flour
1.5 litres (2½ pints) beef stock (low fat, low sodium)
120ml (4fl oz) red wine
2 tbsp dry sherry or cognac
1 bay leaf
½ tsp pepper
4 slices stone-ground wholemeal toasts
90g (3oz) shredded light-style Swiss or Jarlsberg cheese

1. In a large stockpot, heat the oil over a medium-high heat. Cook the onions, garlic and salt, stirring often, for about 10 minutes or until they start to brown. Reduce the heat to medium-low and continue cooking, stirring occasionally, for about 20 minutes or until the onions are very golden and very soft. Add the flour and stir to coat the onions for 1 minute.

2. Add the beef stock, wine, sherry, bay leaf and pepper; bring to the boil. Reduce the heat and simmer for 30 minutes. Remove the bay leaf.

3. Pour the soup into ovenproof bowls. Place the bread on top to fit the bowls and sprinkle with cheese. Bake in the oven at 200°C (Gas Mark 6) for about 15 minutes or until the cheese is bubbly. Then place them under the grill for 30 seconds to brown the tops.

Makes 4 servings.

LIGHTER OPTION: For an even lighter soup, omit the cheese and bread.

STORAGE: You can make this soup through to step 2 up to 3 days ahead. Let it cool to room temperature in the pot; cover and refrigerate. Reheat the soup before continuing with step 3.

HELPFUL HINT: To make your own toasts, place bread slices on a baking sheet. Bake in the oven at 180°C (Gas Mark 4) for about 20 minutes, turning once, or until dried.

MISO SOUP

This is a great starter for an Asian-inspired dinner. Miso is fermented soybean paste that ranges in colour from white to dark brown. The lighter the colour, the milder the flavour. Since miso tends to sink to the bottom, be sure to stir up your soup as you eat it to get its full rich flavour.

900ml (1½ pints) vegetable stock (low fat, low sodium)
450ml (¾ pint) water
1 sheet nori
165g (5½oz) diced firm tofu

120g (4oz) sliced mushrooms
3 spring onions, chopped
3 tbsp miso paste
1 tbsp soy sauce

1. In a large stockpot, bring the stock and water to boil.

2. Meanwhile, tear the nori into small pieces. Add the nori, tofu, mushrooms, spring onions, miso and soy sauce to the pot. Reduce the heat and simmer for about 20 minutes or until the nori and mushrooms are tender.

Makes 4 servings.

HELPFUL HINTS: Nori is used to make sushi rolls. Look for nori, also known as toasted seaweed, in the International section of your supermarket. Some supermarkets sell sushi and will have the ingredients to sell as well. Or look for specialist Chinese or Asian product shops.

You can find miso in health and bulk food stores as well as in Chinese product shops and some specialty food shops.

HAM AND LENTIL SOUP ●

Tinned lentils make this soup quick and easy to prepare, so keep some on hand in the pantry. If you want to make this soup even more green-light, use dried lentils (see instructions at the bottom of this page).

1 tbsp rapeseed oil
1 onion, chopped
60g (2oz) diced celery
2 cloves garlic, crushed
1.5 litres (2½ pints) chicken stock (low fat, low sodium)

2 cans (2 x 410g) lentils, drained and rinsed
180g (6oz) black forest ham, diced
1 red pepper, diced
2 tomatoes, seeded and diced
2 tbsp chopped fresh flat leaf parsley

1. In a large stockpot, heat the oil over a medium heat and cook the onion, celery and garlic for about 5 minutes or until softened. Add the stock, lentils, ham and red pepper; bring to the boil. Reduce the heat and add the tomatoes. Cover and simmer for 20 minutes. Stir in the parsley.

Makes 4 servings.

DRIED LENTIL OPTION: Use 200g (7oz) dried green or brown lentils. Add with the stock, and cover and simmer for about 30 minutes or until tender.

MINESTRONE SOUP

This soup is one of my favourites because it contains both pasta and spinach. Serve it with a sprinkling of grated Parmesan for extra flavour and a few more red pepper flakes to get your blood pumping.

2 tsp rapeseed oil
3 slices back bacon, chopped
1 onion, chopped
4 cloves garlic, crushed
2 carrots, chopped
1 celery stalk, chopped
1 tbsp dried oregano
½ tsp red pepper flakes
¼ tsp each salt and pepper
1 can (400g) plum tomatoes
1.5 litres (2½ pints) chicken stock (low fat, low sodium)
1 bag (300g/10oz) baby spinach
1 can (410g) each red kidney beans and chickpeas, drained and rinsed
120g (4oz) ditali or tubetti pasta
15g (½oz) chopped fresh flat leaf parsley
2 tbsp chopped fresh basil (optional)

1. In a large stockpot, heat the oil over a medium-high heat and cook the back bacon for 2 minutes. Reduce the heat to medium and add the onion, garlic, carrots, celery, oregano, red pepper flakes, salt and pepper. Cook for about 10 minutes or until softened and just about golden.

2. Add the tomatoes and crush them using a potato masher in the pot. Pour in the chicken stock; bring to the boil. Reduce the heat to a simmer and add the spinach, beans, chickpeas and pasta. Simmer for about 20 minutes or until the pasta is tender. Stir in the parsley and basil (if using).

Makes 6 servings.

VEGETARIAN OPTION: Omit the back bacon and use vegetable stock for the chicken stock.

SMOKY BLACK BEAN SOUP

Whenever I make this soup, my husband always asks for more. The wonderful flavour of smoked turkey permeates it. Look for smoked turkey legs in delicatessens.

1 tbsp rapeseed oil
1 onion, diced
2 cloves garlic, crushed
1 jalapeno pepper, seeded and minced
2 cans (2 x 410g) black beans, drained and rinsed
1.5 litres (2½ pints) chicken stock (low fat, low sodium)
1 smoked turkey leg (about 550g (1¼lb)

80g (2¾oz) tomato paste
2 green peppers, diced
1 tomato, seeded and diced
15g (½oz) chopped fresh coriander
60ml (2fl oz) light sour cream

1. In a large stockpot, heat the oil over a medium heat. Cook the onion, garlic and jalapeno pepper for about 3 minutes or until softened. Add the beans, stock, turkey leg and tomato paste. Bring to the boil; reduce the heat and simmer for about 1 hour or until the turkey begins to break apart.

2. Remove the turkey leg and set aside. Pour the soup into a blender in batches and purée it until smooth. Return it to the pot over a medium heat. Add the peppers and tomato and heat until steaming.

3. Meanwhile, remove the meat from the turkey leg and chop; add to the soup. Serve sprinkled with coriander and a dollop of sour cream.

Makes 4 servings.

HAM OPTION: You can substitute smoked ham or hamhock for the turkey leg.

MUSHROOM BARLEY AND BEEF SOUP

A thick, hearty stew-like soup will warm up anyone on a cold winter's night. This is real comfort food for the soul and the belly.

1 tbsp rapeseed oil
240g (8oz) extra-lean minced beef
1 onion, chopped
2 cloves garlic, crushed
450g (1lb) mushrooms, sliced
1 each carrot and celery stalk, chopped
1 tbsp chopped fresh thyme leaves or 1 tsp dried
2 tbsp tomato paste

1 tbsp balsamic vinegar
¼ tsp each salt and pepper
900ml (1½ pints) beef stock (low fat, low sodium)
600ml (1¼ pints) water
120g (4oz) barley
1 bay leaf
1 can (410g) black beans, drained and rinsed

1. In a large stockpot, heat the oil over a medium-high heat and cook the beef until it is no longer pink. Reduce the heat to medium and add the onion and garlic; cook, stirring, for 5 minutes. Add the mushrooms, carrot, celery and thyme and cook for about 15 minutes or until all the liquid has evaporated from the mushrooms.

2. Add the tomato paste, vinegar, salt and pepper; stir to coat the vegetables. Add the stock, water, barley and bay leaf; bring to the boil. Reduce the heat, cover and simmer for about 45 minutes or until the barley is tender. Add the beans and heat through. Remove the bay leaf.

Makes 4 to 6 servings.

CHICKEN OPTION: You can use minced chicken or turkey instead of the beef and use chicken stock instead of beef stock.

NOTE: Mushrooms come in all shapes and sizes. The best for this soup are white or brown button mushrooms, shiitakes, oyster or even portobellos.

CIOPPINO

This Italian-influenced fish stew can be made with whatever happens to be the fresh catch of the day. Adding shellfish such as crab, clams or lobster will make it impressive enough for entertaining.

1 tbsp olive oil	20g (²/₃oz) chopped flat leaf parsley
1 onion, chopped	1 tsp dried oregano
4 cloves garlic, crushed	½ tsp dried basil or 2 tbsp chopped fresh
1 green pepper, chopped	½ tsp red pepper flakes
1 can (400g) diced tomatoes, drained	240g (8oz) mussels, rinsed
240ml (8fl oz) fish or chicken stock (low fat, low sodium)	240g (8oz) cod fillets
120ml (4fl oz) red wine	240g (8oz) large, raw prawns, peeled and deveined

1. In a stockpot, heat the oil over medium heat. Cook the onion, garlic and pepper for about 5 minutes or until softened. Add the tomatoes, fish stock, wine, half of the parsley, oregano, basil and red pepper flakes; bring to the boil. Reduce the heat and simmer for 15 minutes.

2. Meanwhile scrub the mussels and remove the beards; discard any mussels that do not close when tapped. Add the mussels, cod and prawns to the pot; cover and cook for about 5 minutes or until the mussels are open and the cod and prawns are firm. Gently stir in the remaining parsley.

Makes 3 servings.

THAI SHRIMP SOUP

This soup is a huge favourite of my sister's. You can make it with chicken or scallops instead of the prawns. Look for lemongrass in the fresh herb section of the supermarket. Cut the top grassy part off and use the thicker bottom part. Hit the stalk with the back of your knife to release some of the juices before cutting. If you can't find lemongrass, use 4 large strips of lemon rind instead.

900ml (1½ pints) chicken or vegetable stock (low fat, low sodium)
30g (1oz) thinly sliced fresh ginger
2 lemongrass stalks, cut in 1-inch pieces
1 clove garlic, crushed
1 tbsp crushed chili or ¼ tsp red pepper flakes
450g (1lb) large raw prawns, peeled and deveined
120g (4oz) rice vermicelli noodles
120g (4oz) bean sprouts
2 spring onions, chopped
2 tbsp rice vinegar
10g (⅓oz) fresh coriander leaves

1. In a large stockpot, bring the stock, ginger, lemongrass, garlic and chili to boil. Reduce the heat and simmer for 15 minutes. Add the prawns, noodles, sprouts and spring onions; cook, stirring, for about 5 minutes or until the prawns are pink and the noodles are tender.

2. Serve each bowlful with a splash of vinegar and a sprinkle of coriander.

Makes 4 to 6 servings.

NOTE: Ginger and lemongrass are both too tough to eat but provide plenty of flavour.

SALADS

CREAMY CUCUMBER SALAD ●

This salad is reminiscent of veggies and dip. Use as fresh a cucumber as you can find.

1 cucumber
400g (14oz) grape tomatoes, halved
75ml (2½fl oz) light sour cream
75ml (2½fl oz) light mayonnaise
2 tbsp chopped fresh dill or 2 tsp dried
1 small clove garlic, crushed
½ tsp grated lemon rind
1 tbsp lemon juice
½ tsp each salt and pepper
¼ tsp celery seed, crushed

1. Chop off the ends of the cucumber. Cut it in half lengthwise and then cut it into thin slices. Place the slices in a large bowl with the tomatoes and set aside.

2. In small bowl, whisk together the sour cream, mayonnaise, dill, garlic, lemon rind and juice, salt, pepper and celery seed. Pour the dressing over the cucumber mixture and stir gently to coat.

Makes 4 servings.

OPTIONS: This salad is delicious combined with peppers, carrots, radishes, broccoli or cauliflower instead of tomatoes.

BACON SPINACH SALAD
WITH BUTTERMILK DRESSING ●

*The classic combination of bacon and spinach is always a surefire hit.
If you plan to take this salad with you for lunch, pack up the greens and
dressing separately.*

6 slices back bacon
1 bag (300g/10oz) fresh baby spinach
180g (6oz) cooked chickpeas
4 radishes, thinly sliced
60g (2oz) bean sprouts
1 red pepper, thinly sliced
30g (1oz) thinly sliced red onion

Creamy Buttermilk Dressing:
60ml (2fl oz) buttermilk or light sour cream
2 tbsp light mayonnaise
1 tbsp cider vinegar
2 tsp poppy seeds
1 tsp Dijon mustard
½ tsp sweetener
¼ tsp each of salt and pepper

1. In a non-stick frying pan, cook the back bacon over a medium-high heat
until crisp. Let it cool and chop coarsely. In a large bowl, toss together the
spinach, chickpeas, radishes, bean sprouts, red pepper and onion.

2. Creamy Buttermilk Dressing: In a small bowl, whisk together the
buttermilk, mayonnaise, vinegar, poppy seeds, mustard, sweetener,
salt and pepper.

3. Pour the dressing over salad and toss gently to coat. Sprinkle the salad
with the back bacon and toss again.

Makes 4 servings.

MAKE AHEAD: You can make the dressing up to 3 days ahead and store it in
the refrigerator. You can also prepare the salad greens up to 1 day ahead.

ORANGE SALAD OPTION: Omit the bacon from the recipe. Cut the rind
and pith from 2 oranges and slice the fruit into thin rounds and add it to
spinach. Orange Dressing: Omit the buttermilk and add 60ml (2fl oz) of
orange juice.

TANGY RED AND GREEN COLESLAW

Using a vinaigrette in coleslaw makes it low fat and really tangy!
This salad keeps well in the refrigerator.

325g (11oz) finely shredded green cabbage
160g (5½oz) finely shredded red cabbage
2 carrots, shredded
60g (2oz) thinly sliced celery
15g (½oz) chopped flat leaf parsley
120ml (4fl oz) cider vinegar

2 tbsp rapeseed oil
2 tsp sweetener
1 tsp celery seeds
½ tsp salt
Pinch of pepper

1. In a large bowl, toss together the green and red cabbage, carrots, celery and parsley.

2. In a small bowl, whisk together the vinegar, oil, sweetener, celery seeds, salt and pepper. Pour it over the cabbage mixture and toss to coat.

Makes 4 to 6 servings.

STORAGE: Cover and refrigerate for up to 2 days.

CREAMY COLESLAW DRESSING OPTION: Whisk together 60ml (2fl oz) each of plain yoghurt and light mayonnaise, 2 tbsp cider vinegar, 1 tbsp Dijon mustard, 2 tsp sweetener, ½ tsp celery seed and ¼ tsp salt.

MOZZARELLA AND TOMATO STACKS

This salad shows off the colours of the Italian flag and makes a great start to any Italian-themed meal. If fresh basil is unavailable, chop some flat-leaf parsley and sprinkle it over the tomatoes and cheese.

3 small tomatoes, sliced
16 thin slices light mozzarella cheese
16 fresh basil leaves
2 tbsp extra-virgin olive oil

2 tbsp balsamic vinegar
1 clove garlic, crushed
¼ tsp pepper

1. Top each slice of tomato with a slice of cheese and a basil leaf. Pile the slices onto a large platter.

2. In a small bowl, whisk together the oil, vinegar, garlic and pepper. Drizzle the dressing over the cheese and tomato stacks.

Makes 4 servings.

HELPFUL HINT: Buy the small squares (240g/8oz) of mozzarella cheese to get perfect little cheese slices that fit nicely on the tomato slices.

SALADS

COURGETTE SALAD

Here's a new way to use up the courgettes that may be overrunning your garden. Serve this crunchy salad as a side dish with Grilled Rosemary Chicken Thighs (see recipe page 147).

6 courgettes, trimmed
2 red peppers, chopped
15g (½oz) chopped fresh flat leaf parsley
15g (½oz) chopped fresh basil
3 tbsp balsamic vinegar

2 tbsp extra-virgin olive oil
2 cloves garlic, crushed
¼ tsp each salt and pepper
120g (4oz) sliced prosciutto, fat removed

1. Cut the courgettes in half lengthwise and then into 1-cm (½-in) thick slices. In a large pot of boiling water, blanch the courgettes for 1 minute or until bright green and just tender. Drain and plunge the courgettes into cold ice water to chill and stop the cooking process. Drain them again, shaking off any excess water and set aside.

2. In a large bowl, toss together the blanched courgettes, peppers, parsley and basil. In a small bowl, whisk together the vinegar, oil, garlic, salt and pepper. Pour it over the courgettes and toss gently to coat.

3. Cut the prosciutto into thin strips and sprinkle over the salad.

Makes 4 to 6 servings.

STORAGE: Cover with clingfilm and refrigerate for up to 1 day.

HAM OPTION: Substitute black forest ham, smoked turkey or cooked chicken for the prosciutto.

ROCKET AND ROASTED PEPPER PASTA SALAD

Peppery rocket is a perfect match for roasted sweet red peppers. Add some chopped cooked chicken, turkey or ham for lunch for the family. This salad will keep up to three days in the refrigerator.

210g (7oz) whole wheat fusilli or penne pasta
1 large bunch rocket, trimmed
1 jar (200g) roasted red peppers, drained
1 can (410g) artichokes, drained and chopped
4 spring onions, chopped
2 tomatoes, seeded and chopped

60ml (2fl oz) white wine vinegar
2 tbsp extra-virgin olive oil
1 small clove garlic, crushed
1 tbsp chopped fresh thyme or 1 tsp dried
2 tsp Dijon mustard
¼ tsp each salt and pepper

1. In a large pot of boiling salted water, cook the pasta for about 7 minutes or until al dente. Drain and rinse under cold water until the pasta is cool and then place in a large bowl.

2. Tear the rocket into bite-size pieces and add to the pasta. Slice the peppers into thin strips and add them to the pasta along with the artichokes, spring onions and tomatoes.

3. In a small bowl, whisk together the vinegar, oil, garlic, thyme, mustard, salt and pepper. Pour the dressing over the salad and toss to coat.

Makes 4 to 6 servings.

GUACAMOLE SALAD

I've taken all the wonderful flavours of guacamole and put them into this delicious salad. Serve it as a starter for a Mexican-themed dinner, right before your Chicken Enchiladas or Beef Fajitas (see recipes on pages 150 and 152). Roll any leftovers in a wholemeal tortilla or stuff them into a pita for lunch the next day.

2 avocados, chopped	2 tbsp lime juice
1 tomato, chopped	1 tbsp rapeseed oil
½ yellow pepper, diced	Pinch of salt
40g (1⅓oz) diced red onion	120g (4oz) shredded cos lettuce
¼ tsp grated lime rind	1 spring onion, chopped

1. In a large bowl, place the avocado, tomato, pepper, onion, lime rind and juice, oil and salt. Toss gently to combine.

2. Divide the lettuce onto 2 dinner plates. Top it with the avocado mixture and sprinkle with spring onion.

Makes 2 servings.

TABBOULEH SALAD

You often see this salad on the delicatessen counter in the supermarket, but it's very simple to make at home. I've added chickpeas for more fibre. Use flat leaf parsley for the best flavour.

360ml (⅔ pint) water
120g (4oz) bulgur wheat
½ tsp grated lemon rind
2 tbsp lemon juice
2 tbsp extra-virgin olive oil
1 small clove garlic, crushed
½ tsp each of salt and pepper

¼ tsp ground cumin
1 can (410g) chickpeas, drained and rinsed
3 plum tomatoes, diced
Quarter of a cucumber, diced
45g (1½oz) finely chopped flat leaf parsley
20g (⅔oz) finely chopped fresh mint
1 tbsp chopped fresh chives

1. In a saucepan, bring the water to boil and add the bulgur wheat. Cover and reduce the heat to low and cook it for about 10 minutes or until the water is absorbed. Using a fork, scrape it into a large bowl; let it cool.

2. In a small bowl, whisk together the lemon rind and juice, oil, garlic, salt, pepper and cumin; pour it over the bulgur wheat. Stir in the chickpeas, tomatoes, cucumber, parsley, mint and chives until it is well combined.

Makes 4 to 6 servings.

STORAGE: This salad will last up to 3 days in the refrigerator.

AVOCADO AND FRESH FRUIT SALAD

The avocado is a bit of a surprise in this refreshing salad, but it really does go well with fruit, providing a nice colour contrast and a rich creamy texture.

60g (2oz) torn red leaf lettuce
1 avocado, peeled and chopped
1 yellow pepper, chopped
Half a mango, peeled and chopped
Half a papaya, peeled and chopped
1 spring onion, chopped
15g (½oz) chopped fresh flat leaf parsley

Dijon Vinaigrette:
2 tbsp rapeseed oil
1 tsp grated lime rind
1 tbsp lime juice
1 tbsp Dijon mustard
1 small clove garlic, crushed
Pinch of dried thyme
Pinch each of salt and pepper

1. Dijon Vinaigrette: In a small bowl, whisk together the oil, lime rind and juice, mustard, garlic, thyme, salt and pepper and set aside.

2. In a large bowl, toss together the lettuce, avocado, pepper, mango, papaya, spring onion and parsley. Pour the vinaigrette over and toss.

Makes 2 servings.

STORAGE: To take this salad to work, simply pack up the vinaigrette separately from the salad and toss it all together once you're ready to eat. You can make this up to 2 days ahead, if you keep the salad and vinaigrette separately.

MEDITERRANEAN BEAN SALAD

This recipe is a fresh twist on the classic bean salad. It's great for a barbeque or you can pack it away for tomorrow's lunch.

240g (8oz) green beans, trimmed
15g (½oz) sundried tomatoes
1 can (410g) chickpeas, drained and rinsed
1 can (410g) black beans, drained and rinsed
1 yellow or red pepper, diced
120g (4oz) diced red onion
3 tbsp balsamic vinegar or lemon juice
1 tbsp extra-virgin olive oil
½ tsp each of salt and pepper
20g (⅔oz) chopped mixed fresh herbs (such as parsley, mint and basil)

1. In a saucepan of boiling salted water, blanch the beans for 3 minutes. Drain and rinse them under cold water; cut into 2-cm (1-in) pieces. Place the beans in a large bowl and set aside.

2. Meanwhile, soak the tomatoes in 120ml (4fl oz) of boiling water. Let them stand for 10 minutes. Drain them, reserving the liquid. Chop the tomatoes and add them to the beans. Add the chickpeas, black beans, yellow pepper and onion.

3. In a small bowl, whisk together the vinegar, oil, 2 tbsp of the reserved liquid, and salt and pepper. Pour it over the salad and toss to coat. Add the herbs and toss again.

Makes 4 to 6 servings.

STORAGE: Cover with clingfilm and refrigerate for up to 2 days.

BEAN OPTIONS: Use kidney, pinto or Romano beans for the chickpeas and black beans.

CORN OPTION: Add 1 can (200g) of sweetcorn, drained, to the salad for extra colour and flavour.

LEMON DILL LENTIL SALAD

I really love the combination of lentils and chickpeas in this salad, but you can use other types of beans as well, such as red or white kidney beans. For another twist, add a sprinkle of feta cheese and a few olives.

1 tbsp rapeseed oil
1 onion, chopped
1 clove garlic, crushed
300ml (½ pint) water
100g (3½oz) dried lentils
Pinch of pepper
1 can (410g) chickpeas, drained
and rinsed
1 green pepper, chopped
180g (6oz) chopped cucumber
210g (7oz) halved grape tomatoes
20g (²/₃oz) chopped fresh flat leaf parsley
4 lettuce leaves

Lemon Dill Dressing:
2 tbsp rapeseed oil
2 tbsp chopped fresh dill or 1 tsp
dried dillweed
½ tsp grated lemon rind
1 tbsp lemon juice
¼ tsp each of salt and pepper

1. In a saucepan, heat the oil over a medium heat. Cook the onion and garlic for 5 minutes or until softened. Add the water, lentils and pepper and bring to the boil. Reduce the heat and simmer for 30 minutes or until the lentils are tender. Let it cool completely.

2. Meanwhile, in a large bowl, combine the chickpeas, green pepper, cucumber, tomatoes and parsley. Add the cooled lentils.

3. Lemon Dill Dressing: In a small bowl, whisk together the oil, dill, lemon rind and juice, salt and pepper. Pour over the salad and gently stir to coat. Serve the salad on lettuce leaves.

Makes 4 servings.

STORAGE: Cover and refrigerate for up to 3 days.

MAIN-MEAL OPTION: Add some cooked chicken, Black Forest ham or smoked turkey to this salad for a heartier meal.

TOMATO COURGETTE WHEAT GRAIN SALAD

I love wheat grain because it has a wonderful nutty flavour and is very healthy. Cook up a large batch and put the extra in the freezer for another salad or a great addition to soups.

240g (8oz) whole wheat grain	3 tbsp balsamic vinegar
1 courgette, chopped	2 tsp extra-virgin olive oil
15g (½oz) sundried tomatoes	1 clove garlic, crushed
2 plum tomatoes, chopped	¼ tsp salt
15g (½oz) chopped fresh basil	Pinch of pepper

1. In a saucepan of boiling salted water, cook the wheat grain, covered, for about 1 hour or until tender. Drain and rinse them under cold water until cool. Place them in a bowl.

2. Meanwhile, in a small saucepan of boiling water, blanch the courgette for 1 minute. Drain the courgette, reserving the water, and rinse it under cold water and add to the wheat grain. Add the sundried tomatoes to the reserved water and let them stand for 10 minutes or until softened. Drain and chop them finely. Then add them to the wheat grain with the plum tomatoes and basil.

3. In a small bowl, whisk together the vinegar, oil, garlic, salt and pepper. Pour the dressing over the wheat grain mixture and toss to coat.

Makes 4 servings.

STORAGE: Cover and refrigerate for up to 3 days.

BARBECUE CHICKEN SALAD

You can add the chicken to this salad hot off the grill, or barbecue it ahead of time and use it cold. For a packed lunch, stuff it into half a whole wheat pita.

2 tbsp soy sauce
2 tbsp rapeseed oil
2 tbsp chopped fresh coriander
1 tbsp crushed fresh ginger
2 cloves garlic, crushed
¼ tsp Asian chili paste or red pepper flakes

4 boneless skinless chicken breasts
2 each red and yellow peppers
180g (6oz) mixed salad leaves
3 tbsp rice vinegar
¼ tsp salt

1. In a large bowl, whisk together the soy sauce, 1 tbsp of the rapeseed oil, the coriander, ginger, garlic and chili paste. Add the chicken breasts and toss everything to coat it well. Cover and refrigerate for at least 30 minutes or up to 1 day.

2. Meanwhile, cut the peppers into quarters. Place them in a greased grillpan under a medium-high heat. Grill them for about 15 minutes, turning once, or until they start to blacken. Remove them to a plate. Place the chicken breasts in a greased grillpan under a medium-high heat and grill them for about 12 minutes, turning once, or until no longer pink inside. Place them on a plate.

3. Chop the grilled peppers and chicken into bite-size pieces. In a large bowl, toss the chicken and peppers with the mixed salad leaves, and the remaining oil, vinegar and salt.

Makes 4 servings.

STORAGE: This salad will last up to 1 day in the refrigerator.

ROASTING OPTION: You can roast the peppers and chicken instead of barbecuing them. Place the vegetables on a parchment paper–lined baking tray and roast them in a 225°C (Gas Mark 7) pre-heated oven for about 15 minutes. Add the chicken breasts and roast for another 12 minutes or until the chicken is no longer pink inside and the peppers are blackened.

CRAB SALAD IN TOMATO SHELLS

Beefsteak tomatoes are ideal for this dish because their large size will accommodate the filling and because their pulp and seeds are easy to scoop out. Try using shrimps or small prawns, tuna or salmon instead of the crab.

2 pkgs (each 210g/7oz) frozen crab, thawed
4 large beefsteak tomatoes
60ml (2fl oz)light mayonnaise
2 tbsp light sour cream
½ tsp finely grated lemon rind
1 tbsp lemon juice
2 tsp chopped fresh tarragon or ½ tsp dried
Pinch each of salt and pepper
240g (8oz) coarsely chopped cooked chickpeas
½ red pepper, diced
30g (1oz) finely diced celery
15g (½oz) chopped fresh flat leaf parsley
2 tbsp chopped fresh chives
2 tbsp shredded carrot

1. Place the crab in a fine mesh sieve and press out any liquid. Remove any cartilage if necessary and set aside.

2. Cut the top quarter off the tomatoes. Using a small spoon, scoop out the seeds and pulp. Place the tomatoes cut-side down on a paper towel-lined plate.

3. Meanwhile, in a large bowl, whisk together the mayonnaise, sour cream, lemon rind and juice, tarragon, salt and pepper. Add the chickpeas, red pepper, celery, parsley, chives and carrot. Then add the crab and stir to combine. Divide the crab mixture among the tomatoes.

Makes 4 servings.

HERB OPTION: Substitute an additional 3 tbsp chopped flat leaf parsley for the chives and tarragon.

SEAFOOD OPTION: Substitute 350g (12oz) crabstick, chopped finely, or shrimps, or 2 cans (120g/4oz each) tuna or salmon, for the crabmeat.

CRAB MELTS: Omit the tomatoes. Top 4 slices of stone-ground wholemeal bread with the crab mixture and sprinkle with 45g (1½oz) of shredded light-style Swiss cheese. Place them under the grill until melted. This makes a great lunch for 4 people.

PEPPER AND TOMATO BEEF SALAD

Thinly slicing the steak for this salad gives the illusion of a lot of meat while keeping everyone's serving size to the recommended 75–100 grams (3–4oz).

2 tbsp extra-virgin olive oil
2 tbsp red wine vinegar
1 tsp Worcestershire sauce
½ tsp dried thyme leaves or 1 tbsp chopped fresh
½ tsp salt
¼ tsp pepper
240g (8oz) sirloin steak, 2cm (1in) thick
90g (3oz) torn cos lettuce or rocket
1 tomato, cut in wedges
½ each red and green peppers, thinly sliced
Quarter of a cucumber, thinly sliced
15g (½oz) chopped fresh mint or parsley

1. In a large shallow dish, whisk together 1 tbsp each of the oil and vinegar, the Worcestershire sauce, thyme and a pinch each of the salt and pepper. Place the steak in the marinade and turn to coat. Cover and refrigerate for 30 minutes or up to 1 day.

2. Place the steak in a greased grillpan under a medium-high heat and grill for 10 minutes, turning once, for medium-rare. Continue cooking the steak as desired. Place the steak on a plate and cover lightly with aluminium foil for 5 minutes.

3. Meanwhile, in a large bowl, toss together the lettuce, tomato, red and green peppers, cucumber and mint. Whisk together the remaining oil, vinegar, salt and pepper. Drizzle over the salad vegetables and toss to coat.

4. Slice the steak into thin strips and add to the salad. Toss to combine.

Makes 2 servings.

CHICKEN OR SALMON OPTION: Substitute 2 boneless skinless chicken breasts or 2 salmon fillets for the steak.

HELPFUL HINT: To take this salad to work for lunch, simply pack the beef and salad separately. At lunchtime, add the two together.

ASIAN GRILLED TOFU SALAD ●

Marinating and grilling the tofu adds lots of flavour to this salad. Have it with a bowl of Miso Soup (see recipe page 112) for a terrific lunch.

1 packet (350g/12oz) extra-firm tofu
60ml (2fl oz) rice vinegar
3 tbsp soy sauce
2 tbsp chopped fresh coriander
1 tbsp crushed fresh ginger or ½ tsp dried
1 clove garlic, crushed
¼ tsp chili paste or hot sauce
180g (6oz) mixed salad leaves
240g (8oz) grape tomatoes
30g (1oz) bean sprouts
2 spring onions, chopped
2 tsp rapeseed oil

1. Cut the tofu in half lengthwise into 2 pieces. Repeat with each piece to get 4 pieces of tofu and set aside.

2. In a shallow glass dish, whisk together the vinegar, soy sauce, coriander, ginger, garlic and chili paste. Add the tofu to the marinade, turning to coat. Cover and let stand for 30 minutes.

3. Meanwhile, in a large bowl, toss together the salad leaves, tomatoes, bean sprouts and spring onions and set aside.

4. Reserving the marinade, grill the tofu slices in greased grillpan under a medium-high heat, turning once, for about 5 minutes, or until golden brown. Place the tofu on a cutting board and slice it into thin strips. Pour 60ml (2fl oz) of the remaining marinade and oil over the salad leaves and top with the grilled tofu.

Makes 4 servings.

STORAGE: Cover and refrigerate the marinated grilled tofu and salad leaves separately for up to 1 day.

GRILLED PRAWN SALAD

The crisp clean flavour of the mixed salad leaves complements the light spiciness of the shrimp in this salad. This dish is a good choice for entertaining friends for lunch. You can use arugula or baby spinach as well.

180g (6oz) mixed salad leaves
120g (4oz) sliced mushrooms
½ red pepper, thinly sliced
1 tbsp rapeseed oil
2 tsp mild curry paste or powder
2 tsp lemon juice
1 tsp grated fresh ginger
Pinch of salt
350g (12oz) jumbo raw prawns, peeled and deveined

Orange Dressing:
1 tbsp rapeseed oil
½ tsp grated orange rind
1 tbsp orange juice
1 tbsp lemon juice
1 tsp Dijon mustard
1 tbsp chopped fresh mint or ½ tsp dried
1 small clove garlic, crushed
¼ tsp salt

1. In a large bowl, toss together the salad leaves, mushrooms and pepper and set aside.

2. Orange Dressing: In a small bowl, whisk together the oil, orange rind, orange and lemon juices, mustard, mint, garlic and salt; pour it over the salad leaves and toss.

3. In a shallow dish, stir together the oil, curry paste, lemon juice, ginger and salt. Add the prawns and, using your hands, toss the prawns to coat them evenly. Place the prawns in a greased grillpan under a high heat and grill them, turning them once, for 4 minutes or until pink and firm. Add them to the salad leaves.

Makes 3 servings.

SKEWER OPTION: If the prawns you purchase are small enough to fall through your grill, simply skewer them onto a bamboo or metal skewer and grill.

FRYING PAN OPTION: If you don't have a grill, place the prawns in a non-stick frying pan over a medium-high heat and cook for about 4 minutes or until pink and firm.

MEATLESS

INDIAN VEGETABLE CURRY ●

So many wonderful vegetarian dishes come from India. This one has a smooth mild curry flavour, but you can spike up the heat by using a hot curry paste or powder. Serve this with basmati rice.

1 tbsp rapeseed oil
2 onions, cut in wedges
3 cloves garlic, crushed
1 tbsp chopped fresh ginger
1 tbsp mild curry paste or powder
1 tsp cumin seeds, crushed
750ml (1¼ pints) vegetable stock (low fat, low sodium)
2 red peppers, chopped
100g (3½oz) broccoli florets
240g (8oz) green beans, cut into 2-cm (1-in) pieces
1 courgette, chopped
1 can (410g) chickpeas, drained and rinsed
15g (½oz) chopped fresh coriander

1. In a large saucepan, heat the oil over a medium heat. Cook the onions, garlic, ginger, curry paste and cumin seeds for 5 minutes or until softened. Add the stock and bring to the boil. Add the peppers, broccoli, beans, courgette and chickpeas. Cover and simmer for about 15 minutes or until the vegetables are just tender. Sprinkle them with the coriander.

Makes 4 servings.

LENTIL AND RICE FILLED PEPPERS

Stuffed peppers have been around for a long time, and they still make a great meal. You can use any colour of pepper that you like.

300ml (½ pint) vegetable or chicken stock (low fat, low sodium)
150g (5oz) brown rice
¼ tsp salt
¼ tsp dried thyme
1 small carrot, shredded
Half a courgette, shredded

2 tbsp chopped fresh parsley
180ml (6fl oz) low-fat pasta sauce
1 omega-3 egg
2 tbsp grated Parmesan cheese
1 can (410g) lentils, drained and rinsed
4 large red, green or yellow peppers
120ml (4fl oz) water

1. In a saucepan, bring the stock, rice, salt and thyme to the boil. Reduce the heat to low, cover and cook for 25 minutes or until the liquid has been absorbed. Remove the pan from the heat and sprinkle the carrot and courgette on top of the rice; cover and let them steam for 5 minutes or until the carrot is just tender. Spoon the rice into a large bowl, add the parsley and fluff up the rice with a fork.

2. In a small bowl, whisk together 120ml (4fl oz) of the pasta sauce, the egg and the cheese. Pour it over the rice and toss to combine. Add the lentils and toss with the mixture and set aside.

3. Cut the top off each pepper. Remove the seeds and pith. Trim the bottoms of the peppers to make them flat. Set the peppers in a baking dish. Pack each pepper with the lentil and rice mixture. Spread the remaining pasta sauce on top of the peppers. Pour water into the dish and cover with aluminium foil. Bake in a 190°C (Gas Mark 5) oven for 40 minutes. Remove the foil and return the peppers to the oven and bake for 20 minutes or until bubbly and peppers are tender.

Makes 4 servings.

BEAN OPTIONS: Try using beans, like black or haricot, instead of the lentils. Remember to drain and rinse them before using.

RATATOUILLE

Ratatouille is a hearty and pleasing vegetable stew. If there are any leftovers, add more vegetable stock to make a great chunky soup.

1 tbsp olive oil
1 onion, chopped
4 cloves garlic, crushed
Half a fennel bulb, diced
½ tsp each dried basil and oregano

2 courgettes, chopped
1 red pepper, chopped
2 cans (2 x 410g) mixed beans, drained and rinsed
165g (5½oz) diced firm tofu

1 can (400g) diced tomatoes
450ml (¾ pint) vegetable stock
(low fat, low sodium)

180g (6oz) diced aubergine
15g (½oz) chopped flat leaf parsley
¼ tsp each salt and pepper

1. In a large stockpot, heat the oil over a medium-high heat. Cook the onion, garlic, fennel, basil and oregano for 5 minutes or until they start to brown. Add the tomatoes and stock and bring to the boil.

2. Add the aubergine, courgette, red pepper, beans and tofu; return to the boil. Reduce the heat to simmering and cook for about 30 minutes or until slightly thickened and the aubergine is very tender. Add the parsley, salt and pepper.

Makes 4 servings.

SWEET-AND-SOUR TOFU ●

Sweet-and-sour sauce can often be sickly sweet without enough sour or heat to it. This version is well-balanced and offers a great blanket of flavour for tofu, which can be rather bland. You can also use chicken or pork.

1 packet (350g/12oz) extra-firm tofu
1 tbsp rapeseed oil
60ml (2fl oz) unsweetened pineapple juice
60ml (2fl oz) red wine vinegar
30g (1oz) finely chopped red pepper
3 tbsp sweetener
1 tbsp soy sauce
1 clove garlic, crushed
2 tsp crushed fresh ginger
2 tsp cornflour

1. Cut the tofu in half horizontally, then cut each half into 1-cm (½-in) cubes. In a non-stick frying pan, heat the oil over a medium-high heat. Cook the tofu for 10 minutes or until browned. Drain the tofu on a paper towel-lined plate and set aside.

2. In a saucepan, whisk together the juice, vinegar, red pepper, sweetener, soy sauce, garlic, ginger and cornflour. Cook over a medium heat, whisking occasionally, for about 5 minutes or until thickened and bubbly. Add the tofu to the sauce and toss to coat.

Makes 4 servings.

HELPFUL HINT: If extra-firm tofu is unavailable, drain firm tofu and place it on a paper towel–lined plate. Top with another plate and a heavy can as a weight. Refrigerate for 4 hours, checking occasionally to drain any liquid.

FETTUCCINE PRIMAVERA

Primavera means 'springtime' in Italian, and you can use your favourite spring vegetables, such as asparagus, in this pasta. Fortunately, you can get peppers, tomatoes and peas all year, so you can make this dish any time.

60ml (2fl oz) extra-virgin olive oil
320g (10½oz) cubed firm tofu
3 cloves garlic, crushed
¼ tsp red pepper flakes
120ml (4fl oz) vegetable juice
200g (6½oz) chopped fresh asparagus or peas
1 red pepper, thinly sliced

1 carrot, julienned
1 yellow courgette, thinly sliced
180g (6oz) wholemeal fettuccine or linguine pasta
2 plum tomatoes, chopped
15g (½oz) chopped flat leaf parsley
2 tbsp grated Parmesan cheese

1. In a non-stick frying pan, heat 2 tbsp of the oil over a medium-high heat. Brown the tofu on all sides for about 2 minutes and remove to a plate. Reserve the oil.

2. In a large shallow saucepan, heat the remaining oil and reserved oil over a medium heat. Cook the garlic and red pepper flakes for 1 minute. Add the vegetable juice; bring to the boil. Reduce the heat and simmer for 1 minute. Add the asparagus, red pepper, carrot and courgette; cook, stirring, for 10 minutes or until the vegetables are just tender.

3. Meanwhile, in a large pan of boiling salted water, cook the fettuccine for 8 minutes or until *al dente*. Drain and return to the pan. Add the vegetables, tofu and toss to coat. Stir in the tomatoes, parsley and cheese.

Makes 4 servings.

ASIAN GREENS AND TOFU STIR-FRY

The wide variety of Asian greens available in supermarkets these days provides excellent new options for old stir-fries. Shanghai bok choy (Chinese cabbage) is all green while the stalks of baby bok choy are white. Serve this with egg or rice noodles.

4 spring onions
2 tsp rapeseed oil
4 baby bok choy, chopped coarsely
2 Shanghai bok choy, chopped coarsely
2 carrots, shredded
1 red pepper, thinly sliced
60ml (2fl oz) vegetable stock or water
2 tbsp soy sauce

½ tsp toasted sesame oil
1 packet (450g/1lb) firm tofu, drained and cubed
1 clove garlic, crushed
1 tbsp crushed fresh ginger
1 tbsp rice vinegar
1 tbsp sesame seeds, toasted

1. Chop the spring onions, separating the white part from the green. Set the green parts aside.

2. In a non-stick frying pan or wok, heat the oil over a medium-high heat and cook the white parts of the spring onions for 30 seconds. Add the baby and Shanghai bok choy, carrots and pepper. Stir-fry for 5 minutes. Add the stock, soy sauce and sesame oil; bring to a boil. Add the tofu, garlic and ginger. Reduce the heat to medium; cover and cook for 3 minutes or until the vegetables are just tender.

3. Drizzle the vegetables with vinegar and sprinkle with the sesame seeds and reserved spring onions.

Makes 4 servings.

BULGUR WHEAT AND CHICKPEA CHILI

Bulgur wheat takes the place of meat in this satisfying vegetarian chili. You can find bulgur wheat, which is also known as cracked wheat, in health food stores.

1 tbsp rapeseed oil	2 cans (400g each) diced tomatoes
1 onion, chopped	240ml (8fl oz) vegetable stock (low fat,
4 cloves garlic, crushed	low sodium)
2 celery stalks, chopped	2 cans (2 x 410g) chickpeas, drained and rinsed
1 carrot, chopped	120g (4oz) bulgur wheat
1 tbsp chili powder	1 red pepper, chopped
1 tbsp dried oregano	¼ tsp each salt and pepper
1 tsp ground cumin	

1. In a large saucepan, heat the oil over a medium heat. Cook the onion, garlic, celery, carrot, chili powder, oregano and cumin for about 5 minutes or until softened. Add the tomatoes and vegetable stock and bring to the boil. Add the chickpeas and bulgur wheat; reduce the heat and simmer for about 20 minutes or until the bulgur wheat is tender. Add the red pepper, salt and pepper and cook for another 10 minutes or until thickened.

Makes 4 to 6 servings.

RICE OPTION: You can substitute brown, basmati or long-grain rice for the bulgur wheat, but increase the cooking time to 30 minutes.

EASY BAKE LASAGNE

Though cooking the G.I. way usually means starting from scratch, there are some handy convenience products that are low G.I., such as pasta sauce! This lasagne is great for a crowd. All you need to go with it is a tossed salad.

12 sheets of wholemeal lasagne
2 tsp rapeseed oil
1 onion, chopped
1 red pepper, chopped
240g (8oz) mushrooms, sliced
¼ tsp each salt and pepper
1 bag (300g/10oz) baby spinach
240g (8oz) diced firm tofu
240g (8oz) low-fat cottage cheese
2 omega-3 eggs
1 jar (700ml) low-fat pasta sauce
150g (5oz) shredded low-fat mozzarella cheese
2 tbsp grated Parmesan cheese

1. In a large saucepan of boiling salted water, cook the lasagne for about 10 minutes or until *al dente*. Drain and rinse under cold water. Lay the sheets flat on damp tea towels and set aside.

2. Meanwhile, in large non-stick frying pan, heat the oil over a medium-high heat. Cook the onion, red pepper, mushrooms, salt and pepper for about 8 minutes or until golden brown and liquid is evaporated. Add the spinach and cook, stirring, for 2 minutes or until wilted. Stir in the tofu. In a small bowl, stir together the cottage cheese and eggs and set aside.

3. Ladle 120ml (4fl oz) of the pasta sauce into the bottom of a 22 x 33 cm (9½ x 13-in) glass baking dish. Lay 3 lasagne sheets on top of the sauce. Spread one third of the spinach mixture over the top and one third of the cottage cheese mixture. Spread with another 100ml of the pasta sauce. Sprinkle with 40g (1⅓oz) of the mozzarella. Repeat these layers, ending with lasagne sheets on top. Spread them with the remaining sauce and sprinkle with the remaining mozzarella and Parmesan cheeses. Cover with aluminium foil and bake in 180°C (Gas Mark 4) oven for 45 minutes. Uncover it and bake for 15 minutes more or until bubbly and a knife inserted in the centre is hot to the touch. Let the lasagne cool 10 minutes before cutting and serving.

Makes 8 servings.

STORAGE: You can assemble the lasagne and refrigerate it for up to 1 day before baking. You can freeze the baked lasagne whole or in portions and reheat in the microwave.

FISH AND SEAFOOD

CORNMEAL-CRUSTED TROUT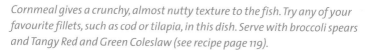

Cornmeal gives a crunchy, almost nutty texture to the fish. Try any of your favourite fillets, such as cod or tilapia, in this dish. Serve with broccoli spears and Tangy Red and Green Coleslaw (see recipe page 119).

150g (5oz) cornmeal
2 tbsp chopped fresh dill or 2 tsp dried dillweed
1 tbsp grated Parmesan cheese
¼ tsp each salt and pepper
Pinch of cayenne
4 fish fillets (trout, cod or tilapia), each 120g (4oz)
1 omega-3 egg, lightly beaten
2 tbsp rapeseed oil

1. In a large shallow dish or pie plate, combine the cornmeal, dill, Parmesan, salt, pepper and cayenne and set aside.

2. Pat the fish fillets dry using paper towels. Brush each fillet with egg and then dip it into the cornmeal mixture, turning to coat both sides well.

3. In a large non-stick frying pan, heat the oil over a medium-high heat. Cook the fish fillets for 3 minutes. Using a spatula, carefully turn the fillets and cook for another 3 minutes or until the fish flakes easily with a fork.

Makes 4 servings.

ALMOND HADDOCK FILLETS

Almonds add calcium to this fish dish. Serve with Lemon Dill Lentil Salad (see recipe page 124), green beans and rice.

75g (2½oz) almonds
15g (½oz) fresh wholemeal bread crumbs
2 tbsp chopped fresh tarragon or 1 tsp dried
1 tsp grated lemon rind
¼ tsp each salt and pepper
1 tbsp rapeseed oil
4 haddock fillets, each 120g (4oz)
Lemon wedges

1. Place the almonds in a food processor; process until the almonds resemble coarse bread crumbs. Put them on a large pie plate or into a shallow dish. Add the bread crumbs, tarragon, lemon rind, salt and pepper and combine.

2. Pat the fillets dry using paper towels. Brush some of the oil over the fish. Dredge them in the nut mixture to coat both sides.

3. In a non-stick frying pan, heat the remaining oil over a medium-high heat. Brown the fish on both sides. Place the fillets on a parchment paper- or aluminium foil-lined baking sheet and roast in a 220°C (Gas Mark 7) oven for about 10 minutes or until the fish just flakes with a fork. Serve with lemon wedges.

Makes 4 servings.

HELPFUL HINT: If you can't find haddock, look for other great whitefish like halibut, cod, tilapia or whiting. You can also try this mixture on salmon or catfish fillets.

TUNA PATTY MELTS

Make these for lunch at home, or omit the cheese and pack them up for the office. Enjoy with the Creamy Cucumber or Lemon Dill Lentil salads (see recipes on pages 117 and 124).

2 cans (100g each) chunk white tuna, drained
1 dill pickle, finely chopped
60ml (2fl oz) light mayonnaise
¼ tsp grated lemon rind
2 tsp lemon juice

2 tbsp finely chopped celery
2 tbsp diced red pepper
¼ tsp each salt and pepper
2 wholemeal muffins
4 slices low-fat Cheddar cheese

1. In a bowl, combine the tuna, pickle, mayonnaise, lemon rind and juice, celery, red pepper, salt and pepper; set aside.

2. Toast the muffins in a toaster or under the grill. Divide the tuna mixture among the muffins. Top with cheese. Place under the grill for 30 seconds or until melted.

Makes 4 servings.

BREAD OPTION: You can serve this tuna mixture on 4 slices of stone-ground wholemeal bread if you like.

SESAME SCALLOP AND BLACK BEAN TOSS

Scallops are rich in protein and zinc, but if they are unavailable, you can use jumbo prawns that have been peeled and deveined.

2 tbsp sesame seeds
240g (8oz) sea scallops
2 tsp rapeseed oil
50g (1²/₃oz) thinly sliced red onion
1 clove garlic, crushed
100g (3½oz) broccoli florets
1 orange or red pepper, sliced

200g (6½oz) cooked black beans
2 tbsp hoisin sauce
60ml (2fl oz) orange juice
½ tsp sesame oil
Pinch each of salt and pepper
15g (½oz) chopped fresh coriander (optional)

1. Place the sesame seeds on a plate. Coat the sides of each scallop with seeds and set aside.

2. In a large non-stick frying pan, heat the oil over a medium-high heat. Brown the scallops on all sides and remove to a plate; cover them to keep them warm. Leave the remaining sesame seeds in the frying pan.

3. In the same frying pan, reduce the heat to medium and cook the onion and garlic for 3 minutes. Add the broccoli, orange pepper, beans, hoisin sauce, orange juice, sesame oil, salt and pepper; cook for about 8 minutes or until the broccoli is just tender. Return the scallops to the frying pan and heat them through. Sprinkle them with coriander (if using).

Makes 2 servings.

TOMATO-TOPPED PRAWNS

Serve these prawns with rice to sop up all the tomato juices. Brighten up your plate with some asparagus and Mediterranean Bean Salad (see recipe page 123).

2 tsp extra-virgin olive oil
1 onion, finely chopped
4 cloves garlic, crushe
15g (½oz) chopped fresh basil
or flat leaf parsley
½ tsp dried oregano
Pinch of red pepper flakes

60ml (2fl oz) dry white wine or chicken stock
2 tomatoes, diced
90g (3oz) coarsely chopped cooked chickpeas
¼ tsp each salt and pepper
240g (8oz) raw prawns, peeled and deveined, or scallops

1. In a non-stick frying pan, heat the oil over a medium-high heat. Cook the onion, garlic, 3 tbsp of the basil, oregano and red pepper flakes for 5 minutes or until they start to become golden. Add the wine and cook for 1 minute.

2. Add the tomatoes, chickpeas, salt and pepper. Cook for about 8 minutes or until the mixture starts to thicken. Add the prawns and cook for 4 minutes or until pink and firm. Sprinkle with the remaining basil.

Makes 2 servings.

HELPFUL HINT: The wine gives a slightly tangy flavour to the sauce. If you use chicken stock, add ½ tsp wine or cider vinegar to the finished sauce before adding the prawns.

GARLIC PRAWN PASTA

Garlic helps keep the heart healthy because it helps to reduce cholesterol and is a great decongestant too. Don't be afraid of the amount of garlic in this dish – the flavour softens as it cooks.

1 tbsp extra-virgin olive oil
6 cloves garlic, crushed
¼ tsp red pepper flakes
120ml (4fl oz) dry white wine or chicken stock
1lb large raw prawns, peeled and deveined
25g (¾oz) chopped fresh flat leaf parsley
1 tbsp non-hydrogenated soft margarine
180g (6oz) wholemeal linguine or fettuccine

1. In a large non-stick frying pan, heat the oil over a medium heat and cook the garlic and red pepper flakes for 1 minute or until the garlic starts to turn golden. Add the wine and bring to the boil. Add the prawns and cook for 5 minutes or until the prawns are pink and firm. Add the parsley and margarine and cook until melted.

2. Meanwhile, in a large saucepan of boiling salted water, cook the pasta for 8 minutes or until *al dente*. Drain and add to the prawn mixture. Toss the pasta to coat it with sauce.

Makes 4 servings.

SALMON STEAKS WITH LIGHT DILL TARTAR SAUCE ●

The marinade and sauce also go well with other fish, such as halibut, bluefish or tilapia. Round out the meal with rice and mixed vegetables.

1 tsp rapeseed oil	Light Dill Tartar Sauce:
1 clove garlic, crushed	60ml (2fl oz) non-fat plain yoghurt
2 tsp grated lemon rind	60ml (2fl oz) light mayonnaise
2 tbsp lemon juice	2 tbsp chopped fresh dill or
1 tsp Dijon mustard	2 tsp dried dillweed
½ tsp each salt and pepper	1 tbsp capers, chopped
4 salmon steaks,	1 dill pickle, finely chopped
each 120g (4oz)	1 spring onion, finely chopped

1. In a bowl, whisk together the oil, garlic, lemon rind and juice, mustard, salt and pepper. Coat the salmon steaks with the mixture; let them stand for 15 minutes.

2. Light Dill Tartar Sauce: In another bowl, whisk together the yoghurt, mayonnaise, dill, capers, pickle and spring onion. Cover and refrigerate it until ready to use.

3. Place the salmon in a greased grillpan over a medium-high heat and grill for 10 minutes, turning once, or until the fish just flakes with a fork. Serve with the Light Dill Tartar Sauce.

Makes 4 servings.

HOISIN ORANGE HALIBUT STEAK PACKETS

The flavours of hoisin sauce and orange go well together and provide a delicious sauce for delicate halibut.

4 baby bok choy, coarsely chopped
240g (8oz) shiitake mushrooms, sliced
1 red pepper, sliced
2 cloves garlic, slivered
2 tsp rapeseed oil
¼ tsp each salt and pepper

2 halibut steaks, each 120g (4oz)
6oml (2fl oz) hoisin sauce
1 tsp grated orange rind
6oml (2fl oz) orange juice
1 tbsp chopped fresh flat leaf parsley

1. In a bowl, combine the bok choy, mushrooms, red pepper, garlic, oil, salt and pepper. Divide the vegetables between 2 pieces of aluminium foil. Top each portion with a halibut steak.

2. In a small bowl, combine the hoisin sauce, orange rind and juice and parsley. Drizzle it over each halibut steak. Cover the fish with another piece of aluminum foil and seal to form packets. Place in a greased grillpan under a medium-high heat, or in a 220°C (Gas Mark 7) oven, for about 20 minutes or until the fish flakes easily with a fork, the vegetables are tender, and the foil packages puff slightly.

Makes 2 servings.

HELPFUL HINT: You can substitute tilapia, sole or haddock for the halibut.

GRILLED PESTO SALMON WITH ASPARAGUS

A little bit of shop-bought pesto can add a lot of flavour to your food. Here it is combined with mayonnaise to form a decadent but light crust for salmon.

6oml (2fl oz) light mayonnaise
2 tbsp chopped fresh flat leaf parsley
1 tbsp pesto
Pinch each of salt and pepper
4 boneless salmon fillets, skin on,
each 120g (4oz)

Grilled Asparagus:
450g (1lb) asparagus spears
2 tsp extra-virgin olive oil
¼ tsp pepper
2 tbsp lemon juice
¼ tsp salt

1. In a small bowl, whisk together the mayonnaise, parsley, pesto, salt and pepper. Spread it evenly over the top of the salmon.

2. Grilled Asparagus: Snap the tough ends of asparagus off and discard. Toss the spears with oil and pepper.

3. Place the fillets and asparagus in a greased grillpan under a medium-high heat. Grill for about 10 minutes or until the fish is firm to the touch

and the asparagus is tender-crisp. Drizzle the asparagus with lemon juice and sprinkle with salt.

Makes 4 servings.

FISH OPTIONS: This pesto mixture is delicious on halibut, tuna or trout.

HELPFUL HINT: Leaving the skin on the fillets helps the fish stay moist and keeps it from falling apart.

LEEK-STUFFED SOLE

A tender leek stuffing gives this fish a burst of flavour. Lemon, olives and tomato add a touch of the Mediterranean.

1 tbsp extra-virgin olive oil
3 leeks, white and light green parts only, chopped
3 cloves garlic, crushed
1 tbsp grated lemon rind
1 tbsp chopped fresh dill or 1 tsp dried dillweed
4 sole fillets, each 120g (4oz)
¼ tsp each salt and pepper
1 tomato, diced
3 tbsp chopped black olives
2 tbsp lemon juice

1. In a non-stick frying pan, heat the oil over a medium heat. Fry the leeks and garlic for about 15 minutes, stirring occasionally, or until softened and golden. Stir in the lemon rind, dill and half each of the salt and pepper. Let it cool slightly.

2. Place 50g (1²/₃oz) of the leek mixture in the bottom of a small casserole dish. Place some of the remaining leek mixture in the centre of each sole fillet; gently fold the fillet over the filling. Lay the stuffed sole in the dish. Sprinkle each fillet with the remaining salt and pepper.

3. In a small bowl, combine the tomato, olives and lemon juice. Sprinkle it over the sole. Bake in a 220°C (Gas Mark 7) oven for about 15 minutes or until the fish just flakes with a fork.

Makes 4 servings.

HELPFUL HINT: To clean the leeks, simply cut the dark green part off and remove any outer layers. Trim the root end. Cut the leek in half lengthwise and rinse under water to remove any dirt. Pat dry and chop.

GINGER SALMON IN PARCHMENT

Cooking in parchment – en papillote – is an easy, healthy way to prepare fish and keeps in all its moisture and flavour. I find that guests enjoy opening their own packages at the table for a 'surprise' dinner.

320g (10½oz) shredded Chinese cabbage
1 red pepper, thinly sliced
120g (4oz) sugar snap peas, halved
4 salmon fillets, skin removed, each 120g (4oz)
60ml (2fl oz) soy sauce
2 spring onions, chopped
1 tbsp crushed fresh ginger
1 clove garlic, crushed
1 tsp sesame oil
¼ tsp pepper

1. Cut four large pieces of parchment paper and fold each in half. Then unfold them and set aside.

2. Combine the cabbage, red pepper and sugar snap peas. Divide the vegetables evenly on one side of the fold of each piece of parchment paper. Place the salmon fillets on top of the vegetables.

3. In a small bowl, whisk together the soy sauce, spring onions, ginger, garlic, sesame oil and pepper. Drizzle it over the fish and vegetables. Fold the empty half of parchment over and fold the edges to seal them. Place the packages on a large baking tray and bake in a 200°C (Gas Mark 6) oven for about 20 minutes or until the fish flakes easily with a fork.

Makes 4 servings.

HELPFUL HINT: If you don't have any parchment, you can still make these delicious packages with aluminium foil.

FISH OPTIONS: Try this recipe with any of your favourite fish, such as halibut, tilapia or snapper.

POULTRY

CORIANDER GINGER TURKEY BURGERS

You can serve these on halves of wholemeal rolls, but they are just as tasty on their own. If minced turkey is unavailable, you can use minced chicken.

1 omega-3 egg, lightly beaten
2 tbsp soy sauce
2 spring onions, chopped
2 cloves garlic, crushed
1 tbsp crushed fresh ginger

15g (½oz) chopped fresh coriander
40g (1⅓oz) crushed wholemeal biscuits or dry bread crumbs
¼ tsp pepper
450g (1lb) lean minced turkey

1. In a large bowl, whisk together the egg and soy sauce. Stir in the onions, garlic, ginger, coriander, crushed biscuits and pepper. Add the turkey and, using your hands, mix it into the egg mixture until it is evenly distributed. Shape into 4 rounds about 1.5-cm (½ -in) thick.

2. Place the burgers in a large non-stick frying pan over a medium-high heat; cover and cook, turning once, for about 15 minutes, or until they are no longer pink inside.

Makes 4 servings.

LEMON YOGHURT CHICKEN

This has been adapted from a recipe that Lenna F. sent to us via e-mail. The yoghurt marinade keeps the chicken breasts juicy and flavourful. Serve them with Lentil and Rice Filled Peppers (see recipe page 170).

240g (8oz) fat-free plain yoghurt
1 tsp grated lemon rind
1 tbsp lemon juice

1 clove garlic, crushed
Pinch each of salt and pepper
4 boneless skinless chicken breasts

1. In a large shallow dish, whisk together the yoghurt, lemon rind and juice, garlic, salt and pepper. Add the chicken breasts and turn them to coat them with the yoghurt mixture. Cover and refrigerate for at least 1 hour or overnight.

2. Remove any excess yoghurt from the chicken and discard. Place the chicken breasts in a greased grillpan under a medium-high heat. Grill them, turning once, for about 12 minutes or until they are no longer pink inside.

Makes 4 servings.

TURKEY AND SUGAR SNAP PEA STIR-FRY

Now that turkey has become more readily available in supermarkets throughout the year, it's not just for the holidays any more. You can use it instead of chicken in any recipe. In this stir-fry, the turkey takes on a great lemony flavour.

450g (1lb) boneless skinless turkey breasts or stir-fry strips
½ tsp each dried sage and thyme leaves
½ tsp salt
¼ tsp pepper
2 tsp rapeseed oil
3 spring onions, chopped

2 cloves garlic, crushed
1 red pepper, chopped
240g (8oz) sugar snap peas, halved
120ml (4fl oz)chicken stock
½ tsp grated lemon rind
1 tbsp lemon juice

1. Cut turkey into bite-size pieces. Sprinkle with half each of the sage, thyme, salt and pepper.

2. In a large non-stick frying pan, heat the oil over a medium-high heat; cook the turkey for 8 minutes or until it is no longer pink inside. Place it on a plate and keep warm.

3. Return the frying pan to the heat and cook the onions, garlic and red pepper with the remaining sage, thyme, salt and pepper for 5 minutes or until softened. Add the peas, stock and lemon rind. Bring to the boil, cover and cook for 1 minute or until the sugar snap peas are just tender. Return the turkey to pan and heat it through. Drizzle with lemon juice.

Makes 4 servings.

GINGER CHICKEN

Ginger adds a wonderful fresh flavour to this chicken dish. The coriander, cumin and turmeric give it a beautiful sunny yellow colour.

2 tbsp rapeseed oil
2 tbsp grated fresh ginger
1 tsp ground coriander
½ tsp ground cumin
½ tsp turmeric
I tsp salt

¼ tsp pepper
675g (1½lb) skinless chicken pieces
200g (6½oz) cauliflower florets
2 carrots, cut into chunks
1 red onion, cut into wedges

1. In a small bowl, combine 1 tbsp of the oil, the ginger, coriander, cumin, turmeric, ¼ tsp of the salt, and a pinch of the pepper. Rub the mixture all over the chicken.

2. Toss the cauliflower, carrots and onion with the remaining oil, salt and pepper. Place the chicken and vegetables on a parchment paper-lined baking tray or roasting pan. Roast in a 220°C (Gas Mark 7) oven for about 35 minutes or until the juices run clear when the chicken is pierced and the vegetables are just tender and golden.

Makes 4 servings.

GRILLED ROSEMARY CHICKEN THIGHS

Chicken thighs are cheaper than breasts but have more flavour and are very tender. If it isn't barbecue weather, bake them in a 200°C (Gas Mark 6) oven for about twenty minutes.

2 tbsp extra-virgin olive oil	2 tbsp chopped fresh rosemary or 2 tsp
2 cloves garlic, crushed	dried rosemary, crushed
2 tsp grated lemon rind	¼ tsp salt
2 tbsp lemon juice	8 boneless skinless chicken thighs
2 tbsp dry white wine	

1. In a bowl, whisk together the oil, garlic, lemon rind and juice, wine, rosemary and salt. Add the chicken thighs and toss them to coat them with the mixture. Cover and refrigerate for 15 to 30 minutes.

2. Place the thighs in a greased grillpan under a medium-high heat. Grill, turning once, for about 20 minutes, or until the juices run clear when the thighs are pierced with a knife.

Makes 4 servings.

HELPFUL HINT: You can use 1 tbsp white wine vinegar or cider vinegar instead of the wine.

HUNTER-STYLE CHICKEN

Ubiquitously known as Chicken Cacciatore, cacciatore meaning 'hunter' in Italian, this dish is a favourite among adults and kids alike. You can use all drumsticks or all thighs if you like.

LIVING THE GI DIET

450g (1lb) skinless chicken drumsticks
450g (1lb) skinless chicken thighs
¼ tsp each salt and pepper
2 tbsp extra-virgin olive oil
1 onion, chopped
4 cloves garlic, crushed

450g (1lb) mushrooms, quartered
1 each red and green bell peppers, chopped
1 tbsp dried oregano
1 tsp dried basil
60ml (2fl oz) dry white wine or chicken stock
1 can (400g) chopped tomatoes

1. Sprinkle salt and pepper all over the chicken pieces. In a large shallow saucepan, heat half of the oil over a medium-high heat and brown the chicken on both sides. Place on a plate.

2. In the same pan, heat the remaining oil over a medium-high heat and cook the onion, garlic, mushrooms, peppers, oregano and basil for about 15 minutes or until the vegetables are beginning to brown. Pour in the wine and stir the vegetables to deglaze the pan. Add the tomatoes and bring to the boil. Return the chicken to the pan. Reduce the heat; simmer for 45 minutes or until the chicken is starting to fall off the bone.

Makes 6 servings.

THAI CHICKEN CURRY

You can use any colour – green, red or yellow – of Thai curry paste in this hot and spicy dish. If you want it hotter, increase the amount of curry paste to 1 tablespoon.

1 tbsp rapeseed oil
2 tsp red Thai curry paste
450g (1lb) boneless skinless chicken breasts, cut into chunks
1 onion, sliced
1 each red and green peppers, thinly sliced
120ml (4fl oz) chicken stock or water
120ml (4fl oz) light coconut milk or light sour cream
2 tbsp fish or soy sauce
15g (½oz) chopped fresh basil or coriander

1. In a large frying pan or wok, heat the oil over a medium-high heat. Add the curry paste and cook for 30 seconds. Add the chicken and stir-fry for 5 minutes. Add the onion and peppers; cook, stirring, for about 10 minutes

or until the vegetables begin to brown. Add the stock, coconut milk and fish sauce; simmer for 10 minutes or until the chicken is no longer pink inside. Stir in the basil.

Makes 4 servings.

VEGETARIAN OPTION: You can substitute 2 packets (350g/12oz each) of extra-firm tofu, cubed, for the chicken, and soy sauce for the fish sauce.

BEEF OPTION: You can substitute 450g (1lb) sirloin steak, thinly sliced, for the chicken, and beef stock for the chicken stock.

ORANGE AND CHICKEN STEW

This dish is based on chicken à l'Orange, which was a popular dish for entertaining in the seventies. It is easy to prepare and has a rich orangey flavour. Serve with rice and a tossed salad.

2 tsp rapeseed oil
450g (1lb) boneless skinless chicken breasts, cut into bite-size pieces
2 onions, chopped
2 cloves garlic, crushed
240g (8oz) mushrooms, sliced
1 tbsp chopped fresh rosemary or 1 tsp dried
1 tbsp chopped fresh thyme leaves or 1 tsp dried
¼ tsp each salt and pepper

2 tsp grated orange rind
2 oranges, peeled and chopped
240ml (8fl oz) chicken stock (low fat, low sodium)
1 bay leaf
1 can (410g) runner beans, drained and rinsed
1 green pepper, chopped
1 tbsp cider vinegar
15g (½oz) chopped flat leaf parsley
2 tsp cornflour
1 tbsp water

1. In a large deep non-stick frying pan, heat the oil over a medium-high heat. Brown the chicken and place on a plate. In the same pan, add the onions, garlic, mushrooms, rosemary, thyme, salt and pepper and cook for 8 minutes or until the liquid has evaporated. Return the chicken to the pan with the orange rind, oranges, stock and bay leaf. Bring to the boil. Cover and simmer for about 30 minutes or until the chicken is no longer pink inside.

2. Add the beans, green pepper, vinegar and parsley; cook for 10 minutes or until heated through. In a small bowl, whisk together the cornflour and water. Stir into the stew and cook until thickened. Remove the bay leaf.

Makes 4 servings.

YELLOW-LIGHT PORK OPTION: You can substitute pork fillet for the chicken.

CHICKEN ENCHILADAS

*I love having themed dinners, and this recipe is perfect for a Mexican fiesta.
Serve these enchiladas with low-fat refried beans and rice for a fun party meal.*

2 tbsp rapeseed oil
2 tsp chili powder
1 tsp ground cumin
1 tsp dried oregano
¼ tsp each salt and pepper
4 boneless skinless chicken breasts, cut into bite-size pieces
2 onions, sliced
1 each red and green peppers, thinly sliced
1 jalapeno pepper, seeded and finely chopped
210g (7oz) drained chopped tomatoes
50g (1²/₃oz) shredded light-style Cheddar cheese
8 large wholemeal tortillas

Toppings:
50g (2oz) grated light-style Cheddar cheese
120ml (4fl oz) low-fat sour cream

1. In a bowl, combine 1 tbsp of the rapeseed oil, the chili powder, cumin, oregano, salt and pepper. Add the chicken and coat it with the mixture. In a non-stick frying pan, heat the remaining oil over a medium-high heat; cook the chicken for about 10 minutes or until it is no longer pink inside. Place on a plate.

2. Reduce the heat to medium and cook the onions, red and green peppers and jalapeno in the same pan for about 10 minutes or until they are tender; set aside.

3. Add the chicken, tomatoes and cheese to the pepper mixture; stir to combine. Divide the filling among the tortillas and roll up. Place in a shallow 22 x 33-cm (9½ x 13-inch) greased baking dish. Cover with aluminium foil and bake in a 200°C (Gas Mark 6) oven for about 15 minutes or until the filling is hot. Remove the foil and bake for another 5 minutes or until the tortillas are crisp. Sprinkle them with the cheese and dollop with sour cream before serving.

Makes 4 servings.

BEEF OPTION: You can substitute 450g (1lb) of sirloin steak, thinly sliced, for the chicken.

PRAWN OPTION: You can substitute 450g (1lb) large raw prawns, peeled and deveined, for the chicken.

MEAT

BEEF AND AUBERGINE CHILI

The addition of aubergine gives this chili a delicious twist.

350g (12oz) extra-lean
minced beef
1 tbsp rapeseed oil
2 onions, chopped
4 cloves garlic, crushed
2 tbsp chili powder
1 tbsp dried oregano

1 tsp ground cumin
2 green peppers, chopped
180g (6oz) chopped aubergine
1 can (400g) diced tomatoes
120ml (4fl oz) tomato paste
1 can (410g) red kidney beans,
drained and rinsed

1. In a large saucepan over a medium-high heat, brown the beef and place on
a plate. In the same pan, heat the oil over a medium heat and add the onions,
garlic, chili powder, oregano and cumin, stirring for about 5 minutes until
softened. Add the peppers and aubergine; cook for 10 minutes or until golden.
Add the tomatoes, tomato paste and beef; bring to the boil. Reduce the heat
and add the beans. Simmer for about 1 hour or until the aubergine is tender.

Makes 4 servings.

EASY MEAT SAUCE

*Half of this recipe served with 175g (6oz) of wholemeal pasta makes a great
dinner for four. You can also use this sauce in lasagne or even eat it on its own.*

350g (12oz) extra-lean
ground beef
1 tbsp rapeseed oil
1 onion, chopped
2 cloves garlic, chopped
1 tbsp dried oregano

1 tsp salt
¼ tsp red pepper flakes
2 cans (2 x 400g) plum tomatoes, puréed
1 each red and green peppers, chopped
4 fresh basil leaves
4 sprigs fresh flat leaf parsley

1. In a deep pan, cook the beef over a medium-high heat for about 8 minutes
until browned. Place it on a plate; reduce the heat to medium. In the same
pan, add the oil, onion, garlic, oregano, salt and red pepper flakes; cook,
stirring, for about 5 minutes or until softened.

2. Add the tomatoes, peppers, basil and parsley and bring to the boil. Return
the meat to the sauce. Reduce the heat and simmer for about 30 minutes or
until thickened.

Makes about 1.6kg (2¼lb).

STORAGE: The mixture can be frozen for up to 1 month.

HORSERADISH BURGERS

The combination of beef and horseradish makes these burgers a hit with meat lovers. For a spicier horseradish flavour, simply smother the top with some more horseradish. Serve with a side of Tabbouleh Salad (see recipe page 122).

1 small onion, grated	¼ tsp salt
1 clove garlic, crushed	2 tbsp wheat bran
2 tbsp horseradish	2 tbsp wheat germ
2 tbsp steak sauce	450g (1lb) extra-lean minced beef
1 tbsp Dijon mustard	2 wholemeal rolls
1 tbsp Worcestershire sauce	4 lettuce leaves
2 tsp dried oregano	1 tomato, sliced
½ tsp pepper	15g (½oz) alfalfa sprouts (optional)

1. In a large bowl, stir together the onion, garlic, horseradish, steak sauce, mustard, Worcestershire sauce, oregano, pepper and salt. Add the bran and wheat germ; stir thoroughly. Let it stand for 5 minutes. Using your hands, mix in the beef until it is well combined.

2. Form the mixture into 4 rounds about 1-cm (½ -in) thick. Place in a greased grillpan or in non-stick frying pan and grill or fry, turning once, for about 12 minutes, or until the burgers are no longer pink inside. Place the burgers on each half of the rolls. Top with lettuce, tomato slices and sprouts (if using).

Makes 4 servings.

BEEF FAJITAS

Here is a restaurant classic that is simple to make at home! Serve the fajitas sizzling from the skillet for great effect.

1 tsp rapeseed oil	½ tsp each ground cumin and
240g (8oz) sirloin steak, thinly sliced	dried thyme
1 tbsp Worcestershire sauce	½ tsp each salt and pepper
Pinch of cayenne	60ml (2fl oz) low-fat pasta sauce
1 red onion, sliced	or low-fat salsa
2 cloves garlic, crushed	4 small wholemeal tortillas
1 each red and green peppers, sliced	60ml (2fl oz) low-fat sour cream
2 tsp chili powder	

1. In a large non-stick frying pan, heat the oil over a medium-high heat. Cook the steak, Worcestershire sauce and cayenne for 5 minutes or until browned. Place on a plate.

2. Return the frying pan to a medium heat and cook the onion, garlic, red and green peppers, chili powder, cumin, thyme, salt and pepper for 8 minutes or until just tender. Add the pasta sauce and cook for 5 minutes. Return the beef to the pan and cook until it is heated through.

3. Divide the meat mixture among the tortillas, dollop with some sour cream and roll up.

Makes 2 servings.

CHICKEN/TURKEY OPTION: You can use boneless skinless chicken or turkey breast instead of the beef.

SERVING OPTION: You can serve the meat mixture over rice instead of filling the tortillas.

BEEFY MEATBALLS

You can use ground pork, veal, chicken or turkey instead of the beef in this recipe. Serve the meatballs on their own or with your favourite low-fat pasta sauce and whole wheat spaghetti.

1 omega-3 egg
40g (1¹⁄₃oz) crushed wholemeal biscuits
15g (½oz) chopped fresh flat leaf parsley
2 tbsp grated Parmesan cheese
2 tbsp wheat germ or wheat bran

2 cloves garlic, crushed
½ tsp salt
¼ tsp red pepper flakes
675g (1½lb) extra-lean minced beef

1. In a large bowl, whisk the egg with a fork. Add the biscuits, parsley, cheese, wheat germ, garlic, salt and red pepper flakes; stir to combine. Add the meat and combine well, using your hands to distribute the ingredients evenly.

2. Roll the meat mixture into 2.5-cm (1-in) balls and place on an aluminium foil-lined baking tray. Bake in a 200°C (Gas Mark 6) oven for 20 minutes or until they are no longer pink inside.

Makes 6 servings or about 24 meatballs.

MINI MEATBALL OPTION: Use a teaspoon measure to make tiny meatballs for your family.

STORAGE: Let the meatballs cool completely. Place them in an airtight container or resealable bag and freeze for up to 2 months.

SPICY BEEF AND BEANS

This dish is mildly spicy and goes well with pasta and Tangy Red and Green Coleslaw (see recipe for 119).

450g (1lb) lean stewing beef
1 tbsp rapeseed oil
1 onion, chopped
1 carrot, chopped
2 cloves garlic, crushed
240g (8oz) mushrooms, sliced
1 tsp dried thyme leaves
½ tsp red pepper flakes
450ml (¾ pint) beef stock

80g (2¾oz) tomato paste
1 tbsp Worcestershire sauce
1 bay leaf
1 can (410g) white beans, drained and rinsed
1 red pepper, chopped
½ tsp salt
¼ tsp pepper
15g (½oz) chopped fresh basil or parsley

1. In a large shallow saucepan, heat some of the oil over a medium-high heat and brown the beef. Place it on a plate and set aside.

2. Return the saucepan to a medium heat and add any remaining oil. Add the onion, carrot, garlic, mushrooms, thyme and red pepper flakes; cook for about 8 minutes or until golden. Add the beef stock, tomato paste, Worcestershire sauce, bay leaf and browned beef and juices. Bring to the boil. Reduce the heat, cover and simmer for 1 hour.

3. Uncover and add the beans, red pepper, salt and pepper. Cover and return to simmer for 1 hour or until the beef is very tender. Remove the bay leaf. Stir in the basil.

Makes 4 servings.

YELLOW-LIGHT LAMB OPTION: You can substitute lamb for the beef.

LAZY CABBAGE ROLLS ●

Making traditional cabbage rolls can be a time-consuming process. If you aren't up to the task but want to enjoy the same great flavour, this is the dish for you. It has all the same ingredients but takes less than half the time to make.

2 tsp rapeseed oil
1 onion, finely chopped
2 garlic cloves, crushed
150g (5oz) basmati rice
350ml (12fl oz) beef or chicken stock (low fat, low sodium)
½ tsp salt
¼ tsp pepper
350g (12oz) extra-lean minced beef
½ tsp fennel or caraway seeds, crushed
½ tsp dried oregano
2 omega-3 eggs
15g (½oz) chopped fresh flat leaf parsley
1 jar (700 ml) low-fat pasta sauce
450g (1lb) shredded cabbage
240ml (8fl oz) water

1. In a small saucepan, heat the oil over a medium heat. Cook the onion and garlic until softened. Add the rice and stir to coat. Pour in the beef stock and half each of the salt and pepper; bring to the boil. Cover and reduce the heat to low; cook for 15 minutes or until the liquid is absorbed. Spoon the rice into a large bowl and fluff with a fork. Set aside.

2. In a non-stick frying pan, over a medium-high heat, cook the beef, fennel, oregano and remaining salt and pepper until browned and cooked through. Add it to the rice mixture; stir in the eggs and parsley until it is all combined.

3. Spread 120ml (4fl oz) of the pasta sauce over the bottom of a 22 x 33-cm (9½ x 13-in) baking dish. Sprinkle one third of the cabbage over the bottom. Spread with half of the rice mixture. Spread with another 100ml of the pasta sauce. Sprinkle with another third of the cabbage and the remaining rice mixture. Finish with the remaining cabbage, packing it down gently. Spread the remaining pasta sauce and water evenly over the top. Cover with aluminium foil and bake in a 180°C (Gas Mark 4) oven for about 1 hour or until the cabbage is tender.

Makes 6 servings.

POULTRY OPTIONS: You can substitute minced chicken or turkey for the beef.

FENNEL OPTION: You can use a combination of ¼ tsp anise seeds, crushed, and ¼ tsp celery seeds, if you don't have fennel.

VEAL PARMESAN

Traditionally, this classic Italian dish is made with breaded, fried veal. I've lightened it up by omitting the bread crumbs and grilling the veal instead. Tuscan White Bean Soup makes a perfect starter for this meal (see recipe page 110).

2 tbsp grated Parmesan cheese
1½ tsp Italian herb seasoning
½ tsp each salt and pepper
450g (1lb) veal escalopes or
leg cutlets

240ml (8fl oz) heated low-fat pasta sauce
15g (½oz) shredded low-fat
mozzarella cheese
2 tbsp chopped flat leaf parsley or basil
(optional)

1. In a small bowl, combine the cheese, Italian herb seasoning, salt and pepper. Sprinkle it on both sides of veal escalopes.

2. Place the veal in a greased grillpan under a high heat. Grill, turning once, for about 5 minutes or until they are no longer pink inside. Place the escalopes in a shallow dish; pour the sauce over the top and sprinkle with mozzarella and parsley (if using).

Makes 4 servings.

FRYING PAN OPTION: If a grill is unavailable, you can cook the cutlets in a non-stick frying pan or in a grill pan with 2 tsp extra-virgin olive oil.

VEGETARIAN OPTION: You can use 1 aubergine, sliced into 1.5-cm (½ -in) thick slices, instead of the veal. Brush the slices with 1 tbsp extra-virgin olive oil then sprinkle them with the mixture. Grill them over a medium-high heat for 20 minutes or until tender. Proceed with the recipe.

HEARTY VEAL STEW

This is one of my favourite recipes to make at the weekend. Long cooking makes the veal melt in your mouth. You can also try beef or pork in this recipe.

675g (1½lb) lean boneless
veal shoulder
2 tbsp wholemeal flour
2 tsp Italian herb seasoning
½ tsp each salt and pepper
2 tbsp rapeseed oil
2 onions, sliced
4 cloves garlic, crushed
1 each stalk celery and carrot,
chopped

750ml (1¼ pint) beef stock (low fat,
low sodium)
10g (⅓oz) dried porcini mushrooms
60ml (2fl oz) tomato paste
1 tbsp Worcestershire sauce
1 can (410g) white kidney beans,
drained and rinsed
120g (4oz) sugar snap peas, halved

1. Trim the veal of any visible fat. Cut into 2.5-cm (1-in) cubes; set aside.

2. In a shallow dish or pie plate, combine the flour, Italian herb seasoning, salt and pepper. Toss the veal in the flour mixture.

3. In a large shallow saucepant, heat the oil over a medium-high heat. Brown the veal in batches and place on a plate. Reduce the heat to medium and cook the onions, garlic, celery, carrot and any remaining flour mixture for 5 minutes or until it all starts to turn golden. Add the stock, mushrooms, tomato paste and Worcestershire sauce. Bring to the boil; return the veal to the pot.

4. Reduce the heat; cover and simmer for about 1 hour or until the veal is tender. Uncover and add the beans and sugar snap peas. Cook for another 15 minutes or until the sugar snap peas are just tender.

Makes 6 servings.

PORK TENDERLOIN WITH
GRAINY MUSTARD AND CHIVE CRUST ●

Pork is a very lean meat and is delicious when paired with mustard. Try different kinds such as Dijon or herb-flavoured mustard for variety. Serve this with carrots, broccoli and rice for a quick but elegant dinner.

1 pork tenderloin, about 350g (12oz)
60ml (2fl oz) grainy mustard
1 clove garlic, crushed

2 tbsp chopped fresh chives or spring onion
1 tsp rapeseed oil

1. Using a sharp knife, trim any excess fat from the tenderloin.

2. In a small bowl, combine the mustard, garlic, chives and oil. Spread it evenly over the pork tenderloin. Place the tenderloin on a small greaseproof paper- or aluminium foil-lined baking tray. Roast in a 220°C (Gas Mark 7) oven for about 18 minutes or until a hint of pink remains inside.

3. Place the pork under the grill for 1 minute to brown; turn and repeat with the other side. Let it stand for 5 minutes. Slice thinly.

Make 3 servings.

HELPFUL HINT: Chop up any leftovers and add to a salad.

VEAL WITH FENNEL AND MUSHROOMS

Veal is a lean and tender cut and is wonderful paired with the aromatic flavour of fennel. Fennel, also called anise, can be found in the vegetable section of your supermarket and has a mild liquorice flavour.

450g (1lb) veal escalopes
I tsp salt
½ tsp pepper
1 tbsp extra-virgin olive oil
450g (1lb) mushrooms, sliced

Half a fennel bulb, thinly sliced
2 tsp dried sage leaves or 2 tbsp chopped fresh sage
120ml (4fl oz) dry white or Marsala wine
15g (½oz) chopped flat leaf parsley

1. Using a meat pounder, pound the veal to 4-mm (⅛-in) thickness. Sprinkle with ½ tsp of the salt, and the pepper.

2. In a large non-stick frying pan, heat half of the oil over a medium-high heat. Cook the veal in batches for 2 minutes per side or until browned. Place on a plate and keep warm.

3. Return the frying pan to the heat and add the remaining oil. Cook the mushrooms, fennel, sage and remaining salt for 15 minutes or until all liquid is evaporated and the mushrooms are beginning to brown. Add the wine and boil for 3 minutes. Pour the sauce over the veal and sprinkle with parsley.

Makes 4 servings.

VEAL PICCATA OPTION: Instead of using wine, use 60ml (2fl oz) lemon juice and ½ tsp grated lemon rind and boil for 1 minute. Add 1 tbsp chopped capers.

PORK TENDERLOIN WITH APPLE COMPOTE

Serve this comforting dish with Brussels sprouts, sliced carrots and some boiled new potatoes tossed in lemon juice and parsley.

1 tbsp Dijon mustard
½ tsp dried sage leaves
¼ tsp dried thyme leaves
Pinch each of salt and pepper
1 pork tenderloin, about
350g (12oz)
1 tbsp rapeseed oil

Apple Compote:
1 tsp rapeseed oil
2 small apples, cored and diced
1 onion, finely chopped
¼ tsp dried thyme leaves
Pinch each of salt and pepper
30g (1oz) currants
2 tbsp apple juice

1. In a small bowl, stir together the mustard, sage, thyme, salt and pepper. Rub the mixture all over the tenderloin.

2. In an ovenproof non-stick frying pan, heat the oil over a medium-high heat. Brown the tenderloin on one side, turn over and place the frying pan in a 200°C (Gas Mark 6) oven for about 20 minutes or until the pork has only a hint of pink inside. Let it stand for 5 minutes before slicing.

3. Apple Compote: Meanwhile, in another non-stick frying pan, heat the oil over a medium-high heat. Cook the apples, onion, thyme, salt and pepper for 5 minutes or until light golden. Add the currants and apple juice; cook for 1 minute or until the apples are just tender. Slice the tenderloin and serve with the Apple Compote.

Makes 3 servings.

PORK AMANDINE

This meal can be ready faster than it takes to set the table! Serve with a big helping of steamed green beans or asparagus.

4 quick-fry boneless pork loin chops
1 clove garlic, crushed
¼ tsp dried thyme leaves
Pinch each of salt and pepper
1 tsp rapeseed oil

60ml (2fl oz) dry white wine
60ml (2fl oz) chicken stock
½ tsp cornflour
2 tbsp sliced almonds, toasted
1 tbsp chopped fresh flat leaf parsley

1. Sprinkle the pork chops with the garlic, thyme, salt and pepper. In a large non-stick frying pan, heat the oil over a medium-high heat. Cook the chops, turning once, for 5 minutes or until browned; put on a plate.

2. Return the frying pan to the heat and add the wine and stock. Bring to the boil and cook for 1 minute. Whisk the cornflour with 2 tsp of water and pour into the wine mixture. Cook, stirring, for 30 seconds. Return the pork chops to the pan, turning occasionally. Sprinkle with almonds and parsley.

Makes 2 servings.

CHICKEN STOCK OPTION: If you don't want to use wine in this recipe, simply use the same amount of chicken stock. Stir in 1 tsp lemon juice to add some tang to the sauce.

HELPFUL HINT: If quick-fry boneless pork loin chops are unavailable, you can use boneless pork loin chops that have been pounded to 4-mm (⅛-in) thickness.

PESTO PORK CHOPS

This is a quick and easy dinner to put on the table during a busy work week.

4 boneless pork loin chops	1 onion, sliced
60ml (2fl oz) pesto	1 red pepper, thinly sliced
¼ tsp each salt and pepper	½ tsp dried oregano
1 tsp rapeseed oil	90ml (3fl oz) chicken stock

1. In a non-stick frying pan, brown the pork chops on both sides over a medium-high heat. Remove to a plate; spread the chops with pesto and sprinkle them with half each of the salt and pepper; set aside.

2. In the same pan, add the oil, onion, red pepper, oregano, and remaining salt and pepper. Cook, stirring, over a medium-high heat for about 4 minutes or until golden. Add the stock and chops, pesto side up. Cover and continue cooking for 5 minutes or until the pork chops have just a hint of pink inside.

Makes 4 servings.

GREEN-LIGHT CHICKEN OPTION: You can use 4 boneless skinless chicken breasts or 8 boneless skinless chicken thighs instead of the pork chops.

PESTO OPTION: Look for sundried tomato pesto in your grocery store and use it in this recipe for a new taste.

APPLE PORK CHOPS

For this dish, choose a cooking apple such as Bramley. Because the sauce is so lovely, be sure to serve these chops with basmati rice.

4 boneless pork loin chops	2 tbsp raisins
½ tsp salt	1 bay leaf
Pinch of pepper	1½ tsp dark treacle
1 tsp rapeseed oil	1½ tsp cider vinegar
2 apples, cored and sliced	¼ tsp dried thyme leaves
1 large onion, sliced	2 tsp cornflour
240ml (8fl oz) water	

1. Trim all the fat from the pork chops. Sprinkle the chops with half of the salt and pepper.

2. In a large non-stick frying pan, heat the oil over a medium-high heat and brown the chops on both sides. Spread the chops with apples and onion. Pour in all but 2 tbsp of the water. Sprinkle with the raisins, bay leaf, treacle, vinegar, thyme and remaining salt. Bring to the boil. Cover, reduce the heat, and simmer for about 45 minutes or until the pork is tender.

3. Remove the lid and whisk together the cornflour and reserved water. Pour it into the frying pan and cook, stirring, for about 1 minute or until the sauce is slightly thickened. Remove the bay leaf.

Makes 4 servings.

APRICOT-SAGE STUFFED PORK CHOPS

These pork chops are wonderful for entertaining. Serve them with green beans and carrots tossed with a touch of extra-virgin olive oil and garlic.

4 thick, boneless pork loin chops
Pinch each of salt and pepper
2 tsp rapeseed oil

Stuffing:
1 tsp rapeseed oil
1 small onion, crushed
2 cloves garlic, crushed
2 tbsp chopped fresh sage leaves or 2 tsp dried
Half a red pepper, diced
60g (2oz) fresh wholemeal bread crumbs
50g (1²/3oz) diced dried apricots
15g (½oz) chopped fresh flat leaf parsley
2 omega-3 eggs
¼ tsp each salt and pepper

1. Stuffing: In a non-stick frying pan, heat the oil over a medium heat. Cook the onion, garlic, sage and red pepper for 6 minutes or until softened. Stir in the bread crumbs, apricots and parsley; remove from the heat. Stir in the eggs, salt and pepper until they are well combined. Set aside.

2. Split open the pork chops almost all the way through, leaving one long side attached, and open them like a book. Divide the stuffing among the chops and fold the other side of the chop over the stuffing. Sprinkle the chops with salt and pepper.

3. In a non-stick frying pan, heat the oil over a medium-high heat. Brown the pork chops on both sides. Place on a greaseproof paper- or aluminium foil-lined baking tray and roast in a 220°C (Gas Mark 7) oven for about 20 minutes or until just a hint of pink remains in the centre of the pork.

Makes 4 servings.

GREEN-LIGHT CHICKEN OPTION: You can use 4 boneless skinless chicken breasts instead of the pork chops.

CHUNKY LAMB AND BEAN STEW

The beans in this dish provide a creamy sauce for the lamb. If you haven't tried this classic combination, it could become a new favourite of your family's.

675g (1½lb) lean boneless lamb
1 tbsp rapeseed oil
2 onions, chopped
2 cloves garlic, crushed
1 tbsp chopped fresh thyme leaves or 1 tsp dried
2 tsp chopped fresh rosemary or ½ tsp dried
½ tsp red pepper flakes
½ tsp each salt and pepper
750ml (1¼ pints) beef stock (low fat, low sodium)
1 bay leaf
1 can (410g) white kidney beans, drained and rinsed
1 tomato, chopped
15g (½oz) chopped fresh flat leaf parsley

1. Cut the lamb into 1.5-cm (½ -in) cubes. In a large shallow saucepan, heat the oil over a medium-high heat and brown the lamb. Remove the lamb to a plate. Reduce the heat to medium and add the onions, garlic, thyme, rosemary, red pepper flakes, salt and pepper. Cook for about 5 minutes or until softened.

2. Add the beef stock, bay leaf and browned lamb to the onion mixture. Bring to the boil; cover and reduce the heat and simmer for 1 hour.

3. Meanwhile, using a potato masher, mash the beans coarsely. Add the beans, tomato and parsley to the lamb; cover and continue cooking for about 30 minutes or until the lamb is very tender and the sauce is thickened. Remove the bay leaf.

Makes 4 servings.

ARTICHOKE AND PORK STEW

Tinned artichokes need a good rinse before using to remove the brine flavour. Serve this dish with rice and mixed salad leaves tossed with balsamic vinegar and pepper.

675g (1½lb) boneless pork loin chops
2 tbsp wholemeal flour
1 tsp ground cumin
¼ tsp each turmeric and ground coriander
¼ tsp salt
Pinch each of cinnamon and cloves
2 tbsp rapeseed oil (approx)
240ml (8fl oz) chicken stock (low fat, low sodium) or water
2 onions, chopped
2 cloves garlic, crushed
1 carrot, chopped
1 green pepper, chopped
1 can (400g) chopped tomatoes
1 can (410g) artichoke hearts, drained and rinsed and quartered
150g (5oz) frozen peas

1. Cut the pork chops into 1.5-cm- (½-in)thick strips and set aside. In a shallow dish or pie plate, combine the flour, cumin, turmeric, coriander, salt, cinnamon and cloves; toss the pork strips in the flour mixture.

2. In a large shallow saucepan, heat 1 tbsp of the oil over a medium-high heat; brown the pork in batches, adding more oil if necessary. Remove the pork and put on a plate. Add the stock to the pan and scrape up the brown bits, stirring constantly. Add the onion, garlic, carrot and pepper; cook for 5 minutes. Add the tomatoes and bring to the boil. Return the meat and juices to the pan; reduce the heat, cover and simmer for about 1 hour or until the pork is tender.

3. Add the artichokes and peas and cook, uncovered, for 15 minutes or until slightly thickened.

Makes 6 servings.

MEAT

SNACKS

DRIED CHICKPEAS

This is an addictive snack with all the crunch and saltiness of chips and pretzels but without the fat!

2 cans (2 x 410g) chickpeas, drained and rinsed
2 tbsp extra-virgin olive oil or rapeseed oil
½ tsp salt
Pinch of cayenne

1. In a large bowl, toss the chickpeas with the oil, salt and cayenne. Spread them onto large baking sheet in a single layer.

2. Bake them in a 200°C (Gas Mark 6) oven, shaking the pan a couple of times during cooking, for about 45 minutes, or until golden. Leave to cool.

Makes about 675g (1½lb).

HELPFUL HINT: You can add more salt or other spices if you would like to change the flavour of the chickpeas.

SAGE AND TOMATO WHITE BEAN DIP

I like to serve this at parties with vegetables and whole wheat pita crisps. It's also great smeared over a turkey sandwich.

2 tbsp chopped sundried tomatoes
60ml (2fl oz) boiling water
1 can (410g) white kidney beans, drained and rinsed
2 tbsp extra-virgin olive oil
½ tsp salt
Pinch of pepper
1 tbsp chopped fresh sage leaves or ½ tsp dried
1 small clove garlic, crushed

1. Place the tomatoes in boiling water; let them stand for 10 minutes. Drain them and reserve the water.

2. In a food processor, purée together the beans, tomatoes, oil, salt and pepper and 2 tbsp of the reserved water until smooth. Pulse in the sage and garlic.

Makes 240g (8oz).

STORAGE: Keep in airtight container, refrigerated, for up to 2 weeks.

FRESH FRUIT BOWL ●

Keep this in the fridge and scoop up bowlfuls for an afternoon snack or after-dinner pick-me-up.

2 oranges

2 kiwis, peeled and sliced

2 nectarines, pitted and sliced

1 star fruit, sliced (optional)

210g (7oz) halved strawberries

120g (4oz) red or green seedless grapes

150g (5oz) blueberries or raspberries

1 tbsp sweetener

2 tsp lemon juice

Pinch of ground ginger

1. Using a serrated knife, cut both ends off the oranges as well as all the peel and pith. Over a large bowl, cut the orange sections between the membranes. Into another small bowl, squeeze any juice from the reserved membranes and set aside.

2. Add the kiwis, nectarines, star fruit (if using), strawberries, grapes and blueberries to the oranges. Toss to combine.

3. Add the sweetener, lemon juice and ginger to the reserved orange juice. Pour it over fruit.

Makes 4 servings.

STORAGE: Cover and refrigerate for up to 2 days.

SERVING OPTION: You can sprinkle the fruit with sliced almonds and serve with a dollop of yoghurt, if desired.

ROASTED RED PEPPER HUMMUS ●

Serve this as a dip with raw veggies or as a spread for sandwiches or hamburgers. You could also enjoy it on its own in half a whole wheat pita with tomatoes and cucumber slices.

1 can (410g) chickpeas, drained and rinsed

60g (2oz) chopped roasted red peppers

30g (1oz) tahini

½ tsp ground cumin

½ tsp salt

2 tbsp extra-virgin olive oil

2 tbsp water

1 tbsp lemon juice

1 small clove garlic, crushed

1. In a food processor, pulse together the chickpeas, peppers, tahini, cumin and salt. With the food processor running, add the oil and water until it is very smooth. Pulse in the lemon juice and garlic.

Makes about 675g (1½ lb).

SUNDRIED TOMATO VERSION: Omit the roasted red peppers. Use 15g (½oz) chopped sundried tomatoes that have been rehydrated in hot water and drained.

ROASTED VEGETABLE HUMMUS: Omit the roasted red peppers. Use 120g (4oz) chopped roasted vegetables.

STORAGE: Keep in an airtight container, refrigerated, for up to 2 weeks.

HELPFUL HINT: Tahini is a sesame seed paste that you can find in most supermarkets. You can also find it in health food shops. It adds a great nutty flavour to the hummus.

BAKED APPLE

I love this recipe because it's so quick and easy and you can double or triple it as need be. Baked apples make a delicious sweet snack – and they're also very healthy. You could even have this for breakfast.

1 apple
3 tbsp Muesli (see recipe page 102)
1 tbsp non-hydrogenated soft margarine
1 tbsp raisins
2 tsp sweetener
Pinch of cinnamon or nutmeg

1. Using an apple corer or melon baller, remove the core from the apple. Place the apple on a small plate or in a bowl.

2. Combine the Muesli, margarine, raisins and sweetener and stuff into the centre of the apple. Any excess should be pressed on top. Sprinkle the apple with cinnamon. Cover loosely with clingfilm. Microwave on High for about 3 minutes or until the apple is tender when pierced with a knife.

Makes 1 serving.

HELPFUL HINT: Microwave cooking times will vary depending on the wattage of your microwave. You can check the apple halfway through and determine how much longer it needs to bake.

PEAR OPTION: Omit the apple and use a firm, ripe Bartlett or Bosc pear. It will take less time to cook the pear.

WHOLEMEAL SCONES

Have these scones with a hot cup of tea in the afternoon. The sweet fruit version makes a wonderful breakfast treat when spread with a little sugar-free fruit spread.

180g (6oz) wholemeal flour
75g (2½oz) oat bran
3 spring onions, chopped
3 tbsp flax or sunflower seeds
2 tsp baking powder
2 tsp sweetener

½ tsp salt
¼ tsp nutmeg
50g (1²/₃oz) non-hydrogenated soft margarine
150ml (¼ pint) skimmed milk
1 egg white

1. In a large bowl, combine the flour, oat bran, onions, flax seeds, baking powder, sweetener, salt and nutmeg. Using your fingers, rub the margarine into the flour mixture to combine it. Add the milk and toss with a fork to make a soft dough.

2. Place the dough onto a floured surface and knead gently about 5 times. Pat the dough out to a 1.5-cm (½-in) thickness. Cut the dough into 8 squares, or use a scone cutter to cut the scones out. Place them on a baking tray and brush the tops with the egg white. Bake in a 220°C (Gas Mark 7) oven for about 12 minutes or until golden on the bottom.

Makes 8 scones.

Sweet Fruit Option: Omit the spring onions and flax seeds. Increase the sweetener to 2 tbsp and add 90g (3oz) chopped dried apricots, raisins or dried cranberries.

ORANGE BRAN MUFFINS

Ruth enjoys making these muffins for Rick and many of their friends. Though the recipe calls for a whole orange, the sweetener removes the bitterness of the rind. Use a navel orange, which has no seeds and is very juicy.

1 orange, unpeeled
180ml (6fl oz) skimmed milk
120ml (4fl oz) orange juice
50g (1²/₃oz) non-hydrogenated soft margarine
1 omega-3 egg
1 tsp vanilla
240g (8oz) wholemeal flour

30g (1oz) wheat bran
sweetener equivalent to 60g (2oz) sugar
1 tsp baking powder
1 tsp bicarbonate of soda
1 tsp cinnamon
Pinch of salt

1. Cut the orange into 8 wedges. Place them in a food processor bowl and pulse until finely chopped or almost puréed. Add the milk, orange juice, margarine, egg and vanilla; purée until combined.

2. In a large bowl, combine the flour, bran, sweetener, baking powder, baking soda, cinnamon and salt. Pour the orange mixture over the flour mixture and stir until just combined. Divide the batter among 12 lined or greased muffin cups. Bake in a 200°C (Gas Mark 6) oven for about 20 minutes or until golden and firm to the touch.

Makes 12 muffins.

STORAGE: These muffins can be kept at room temperature for about 2 days or frozen for up to 1 month.

CRANBERRY CINNAMON BRAN MUFFINS

My aunt Carmen is a nurse and likes to make big batches of these muffins to bring to her co-workers on the nightshift. They are very nutritious, with a high fibre content, and have a great cinnamon flavour.

50g (1²/₃oz) wheat bran
30g (1oz) All-Bran or 100% Bran cereal
¼ tsp salt
120ml (4fl oz) boiling water
240ml (8fl oz) skimmed milk
165g (5½oz) dried cranberries
sweetener equivalent to 80g (2²/₃oz) of sugar

1 egg
60ml (2fl oz) rapeseed oil
150g (5oz) wholemeal flour
1¼ tsp bicarbonate of soda
1 tsp cinnamon

1. In a bowl, combine the bran, cereal and salt. Pour the boiling water over and stir to combine. Stir in the milk and cranberries and set aside.

2. In another bowl, whisk together the sweetener, egg and oil. Stir into the bran mixture.

3. In a large bowl, stir together the flour, baking soda and cinnamon. Pour the bran mixture over the flour mixture and stir until just combined. Divide the batter among 12 lined or greased muffin cups. Bake in a 190°C (Gas Mark 5) oven for about 20 minutes or until a skewer inserted in the centre comes out clean.

Makes 12 muffins.

STORAGE: These muffins can be kept at room temperature for about 2 days or frozen for up to 1 month. Wrap each muffin individually before freezing to help prevent freezer burn. Then place them in a resealable plastic bag or an airtight container.

LEMON BLUEBERRY MUFFINS

Lemon and blueberries have a natural affinity for each other. You can wrap these muffins individually in clingfilm and store them in large resealable plastic bags in the freezer. When you feel like having one, let it come to room temperature or pop it in the microwave for that fresh-out-of-the-oven taste.

180g (6oz) wholemeal flour
30g (1oz) wheat bran
sweetener equivalent to
120g (4oz) sugar
1 tbsp baking powder
½ tsp salt

240ml (8fl oz) skimmed milk
1 omega-3 egg
50g (1²/₃oz) non-hydrogenated soft
margarine, melted, or rapeseed oil
1 tbsp grated lemon rind
140g (4½oz) fresh or frozen blueberries

1. In a large bowl, combine the flour, bran, sweetener, baking powder and salt. In a small bowl, whisk together the milk, egg, margarine and lemon rind. Pour the milk mixture over the flour mixture and stir just until combined. Stir in the blueberries.

2. Divide the batter among 9 lined or greased muffin cups. Fill the remaining empty muffin cups with a bit of water to prevent burning. Bake in a 190°C (Gas Mark 5) oven for about 20 minutes or until golden and firm to the touch.

Makes 9 muffins.

HELPFUL HINT: If using frozen blueberries, do not thaw. Use them directly.

STORAGE: These muffins can be kept at room temperature for about 2 days or frozen for up to 3 weeks.

APPLE RAISIN BREAD

A slice of this bread makes a delicious afternoon snack. You can also toast it and top it with a little margarine. Keep this bread wrapped in clingfilm and aluminium foil to lengthen its storage. It freezes well for up to one month.

150g (5oz) wholemeal flour
30g (1oz) wheat bran
sweetener equivalent to
120g (4oz) sugar
2 tsp cinnamon
1 tsp baking powder
½ tsp baking soda
¼ tsp nutmeg
¼ tsp salt

2 apples, cored and diced
50g (1²/₃oz) raisins
40g (1¹/₃oz) chopped pecans or
almonds (optional)
240ml (8fl oz) buttermilk
2 omega-3 eggs
60ml (2fl oz) rapeseed oil
2 tbsp sweetener (optional)

1. In a large bowl, combine the flour, bran, sweetener, cinnamon, baking powder, baking soda, nutmeg and salt. Toss in the apples, raisins and pecans (if using) and coat with the mixture.

2. Whisk together the buttermilk, eggs and oil. Pour this over the flour mixture and stir until just combined. Pour the batter into a 22 x 15 cm (9½ x 5-in) greased loaf pan. Sprinkle the top with brown sweetener (if using). Bake in a 180°C (Gas Mark 4) oven for about 45 minutes or until golden and a skewer inserted in the centre comes out clean. Let it cool on a rack.

Makes 1 loaf, or 12 slices.

HELPFUL HINT: You don't have buttermilk in your refrigerator? No problem, you can make soured milk, which is a perfect substitute. Add 1 tbsp lemon juice or white vinegar to 240ml (8fl oz) skimmed milk. Let it stand for a couple of minutes. Stir, and presto – you have soured milk.

DESSERTS

POACHED PEARS

Poaching pears in fruit juice adds to their sweetness and gives them a richer flavour. Serve them with a dollop of Yoghurt Cheese (recipe page 101) or low-fat, no-added-sugar ice cream.

450ml (¾ pint) pear juice
4 black peppercorns
2 whole cloves
1 cinnamon stick
2 pears, cored and quartered

1. In a saucepan, bring the juice, peppercorns, cloves and cinnamon stick to the boil. Reduce the heat to simmer and add the pears. Simmer for about 10 minutes or until the pears are tender when pierced with a knife. Place them in a bowl.

2. Boil the juice mixture again for 3 minutes. Strain over the pears.

Makes 2 servings.

HELPFUL HINT: Look for ripe pears by picking them up and pressing gently on their skin. If a pear yields slightly and smells fresh and ripe, then that's the one you want to bring home.

BASMATI RICE PUDDING

Here is quintessential comfort food to warm the heart and soul. Try serving this with other favourite fruits such as strawberries or plums.

750ml (1¼ pint) skimmed milk
120g (4oz) basmati rice
sweetener equivalent to
60g (2oz) sugar

1 tsp vanilla essence
¼ tsp ground cardamom or cinnamon
2 peaches or nectarines, peeled
and sliced thinly

1. In a heavy saucepan, bring the milk and rice to the boil over a medium heat. Reduce the heat to low; stir, cover and cook for about 30 minutes or until most of the milk is absorbed. Stir in the sweetener, vanilla and cardamom.

2. Spoon into 4 custard cups and top with sliced peaches.

Makes 4 servings.

BERRY CRUMBLE

This is one of Ruth's favourite green-light desserts. Though it's best made with fresh berries during the summer, it's also lovely with frozen fruit.

675g (1½lb) fresh or frozen
berries, such as raspberries,
blackberries, blueberries and
sliced strawberries
1 large apple, cored and chopped
2 tbsp wholemeal flour
2 tbsp sweetener
½ tsp cinnamon

Topping:
120g (4oz) large-flake oats
60g (2oz) chopped pecans or walnuts
sweetener equivalent to 60g (2oz) sugar
50g (1²/³oz) non-hydrogenated soft
margarine, melted
1 tsp cinnamon

1. In a 20-cm (8-in) square baking dish, combine the berries and apple. In a bowl, combine the flour, sweetener and cinnamon. Sprinkle this over the fruit and toss gently.

2. Topping: In a bowl, combine the oats, pecans, brown sweetener, margarine and cinnamon. Sprinkle this over the fruit mixture. Bake in a 180°C (Gas Mark 4) oven for about 30 minutes or until the fruit is tender and the top is golden.

Makes 6 servings.

MICROWAVE OPTION: Prepare as above and microwave on High for about 6 minutes or until fruit is tender. The top won't get golden or crisp in the microwave.

GLAZED APPLE TART

This tart is worthy enough to serve to company and is especially pretty made with red-skinned apples.

150g (5oz) whole almonds
40g (1¹/₃oz) dried wholemeal biscuit or bread crumbs
1 tsp cinnamon
2 egg whites, lightly beaten
120ml (4fl oz) unsweetened apple sauce*

1 omega-3 egg
2 tbsp sweetener
¼ tsp almond extract
2 apples, cored
2 tbsp low sugar apricot or peach jam**

1. Place the almonds on a baking sheet and toast in a 180°C (Gas Mark 4) oven for about 10 minutes or until fragrant. Let them cool.

2. In a food processor, grind the almonds finely and place in a bowl. Add the bread crumbs and ½ tsp of the cinnamon; toss to combine. Add the egg whites and stir to combine. Press the mixture into the bottom and up the sides of a 20-cm (8-in) pie dish. Bake in a 180°C (Gas Mark 4) oven for about 10 minutes or until firm. Let it cool.

3. In a bowl, whisk together the apple sauce, egg, sweetener, remaining cinnamon and almond extract. Spread this over the bottom of the crust.

4. Cut the apples in half and cut thin half-moon-shaped slices. Place them in concentric circles over the apple sauce mixture. Bake in a 200°C (Gas Mark 6) oven for about 15 minutes or until the apples are tender when pierced with a knife. Brush the top with jam. Let the tart cool on a rack.

* See 'Apples' on page 175.
** Look for jams where fruit not sugar is the first ingredient listed.

Makes 6 servings.

BAKED CHOCOLATE MOUSSE

Seemingly sinful, this mousse is dense and rich. Make it on the weekend to enjoy throughout the week.

240ml (8fl oz) skimmed milk
90g (3oz) unsweetened chocolate, chopped
3 omega-3 eggs

sweetener equivalent to 240g (8oz) sugar
2 tsp vanilla essence

1. In a saucepan, heat the milk over a medium heat until it is steaming. Whisk in the chocolate until it has melted.

2. In a bowl, whisk together the eggs, sweetener and vanilla. Gradually whisk the milk mixture into the egg mixture until they are combined. Pour

it into 4 ramekins. Place the cups in a 20-cm (8-in) baking dish. Fill the dish with boiling water halfway up around the ramekins.

3. Bake them in a 160°C (Gas Mark 3) oven for about 25 minutes or until a knife inserted in the centre comes out creamy.

Makes 4 servings.

HELPFUL HINT: Let them cool completely before refrigerating so no water droplets will form on the surface.

STORAGE: Cover them with clingfilm and refrigerate for up to 1 week.

ALMOND BRAN HAYSTACKS ●

These biscuits are best the day they are baked. After that they tend to lose their crispness, though they still taste yummy. Enjoy them with a cup of decaffeinated coffee or skimmed milk.

2 egg whites	75g (2½oz) All-Bran or 100% Bran cereal
¼ tsp cream of tartar	45g (1½oz) chopped almonds, toasted
sweetener equivalent to	1 tbsp vanilla essence
80g (2²/₃oz) sugar	¼ tsp almond extract

1. In a large bowl, beat the egg whites and cream of tartar until soft peaks form. Gradually add the sweetener and beat until stiff peaks form. Fold in the cereal, almonds, vanilla and almond extract until it is combined.

2. Drop the batter by tablespoonfuls onto a greaseproof paper-lined baking tray. Bake in a 160°C (Gas Mark 3) oven for about 15 minutes or until they are lightly browned and firm to the touch. Let them cool completely.

Makes about 18 biscuits.

STORAGE: Keep in an airtight container for up to 5 days. These do not freeze well.

APPLE PIE COOKIES

These cookies combine all the flavours of a traditional apple pie and have a texture similar to that of a soft granola bar. A great snack!

100g (3½oz) large-flake oatmeal	sweetener equivalent to
90g (3oz) wholemeal flour	80g (2²/₃oz) of sugar
1 tsp cinnamon	2 omega-3 eggs
½ tsp baking powder	2 tsp vanilla essence
Pinch each of nutmeg and salt	1 apple, cored and finely diced
240ml (8fl oz) unsweetened apple sauce/purée*	

1. In a large bowl, combine the oatmeal, flour, cinnamon, baking powder, nutmeg and salt. In another bowl, whisk together the apple sauce, sweetener, eggs and vanilla essence. Pour this over the oatmeal mixture and stir to combine. Add the apple and stir to distribute evenly.

2. Drop heaped tablespoonfuls of the mixture onto a greaseproof paper-lined baking tray. Bake in a 140°C (Gas Mark 1) oven for about 25 minutes or until firm and lightly golden. Let them cool completely.

* See 'Apples' on page 175.

Makes about 18 cookies.

STORAGE: Keep in an airtight container for up to 3 days or freeze for up to 2 weeks.

PECAN BROWNIES ●

Brownies, you ask? That's right. These are packed with fibre and are absolutely scrumptious, so get baking!

1 can (410g) white or red kidney or black beans, drained and rinsed
120ml (4fl oz) skimmed milk
2 omega-3 eggs
50g (1²/₃oz) soft non-hydrogenated margarine, melted
1 tbsp vanilla essence
sweetener equivalent to 180g (6oz) sugar
60g (2oz) wholemeal flour
60g (2oz) unsweetened cocoa powder
1 tsp baking powder
Pinch of salt
75g (2½oz) chopped toasted pecans

1. In a food processor, purée the beans until coarse. Add in the milk, eggs, margarine and vanilla and purée until smooth, scraping down the sides a few times. Set it aside.

2. In a large bowl, combine the sweetener, flour, cocoa, baking powder and salt. Pour the bean mixture over the flour mixture. Stir to combine. Scrape the mixture into a greaseproof paper-lined 20-cm (8-in) square baking pan, smoothing the top. Sprinkle it with pecans.

3. Bake in a 180°C (Gas Mark 4) oven for about 18 minutes or until a skewer inserted into the centre comes out clean. Allow to cool on a rack.

Makes 16 brownies.

STORAGE: Cover these brownies with clingfilm or store them in an airtight container for up to 4 days. They can also be frozen for up to 2 weeks.

Appendix I
Green-Light Glossary

The following is a summary of the most popular green-light foods.

Almonds
This is the perfect nut in that it has the highest monounsaturated fat (good fat) content of any nut, and recent research indicates that almonds can significantly lower LDL, or bad, cholesterol. They are also excellent sources of Vitamin E, fibre and protein. They provide a great boost to the beneficial fat content of your meals, especially at breakfast or in salads and desserts. Because all nuts are high in calories, use them in moderation.

Apples
A real staple. Eat them fresh for a snack or dessert. Unsweetened apple sauce (e.g. Clearspring Organic Apple Puree) goes well with cereals, or with cottage cheese as a snack.

Barley
An excellent supplement to soups.

Beans
If there's one food you can never get enough of, it's beans, or legumes. This perfect green-light food is high in protein and fibre and can supplement nearly every meal. Make bean salads or just add beans to any salad. Add them to soups, use them to replace some of the meat in casseroles or put them in a meat loaf. You can serve them as a side vegetable or as an alternative to potatoes, rice or pasta. A wide range of tinned and frozen beans is available. Exercise some caution with baked beans, as the sauce can be high-fat and high-calorie. Check labels for low-fat, low-sugar versions and watch the size of your serving. Beans have a well-deserved reputation for creating 'wind', so be patient until your body adapts – as it will – to your increased consumption.

Bread
Most breads are red-light except for 100% stone-ground wholemeal or coarse whole grain breads that have around 2½ to 3 grams of fibre per slice (not serving). Check labels carefully as the bread industry likes to confuse the unwary. The wording to look for on packages is '100% stone-ground'. Most bread is made from flour that is ground by steel rollers, which strip away the bran coating, leaving a very fine powder ideal for producing light, fluffy breads and pastries. Conversely, stone-ground flour is coarser and retains more of its bran coating, so it is digested more slowly in your stomach. Even with bread made from whole grains, you have to watch your quantity. Have only one slice per meal.

Cereals

Use only large-flake porridge oats, oat bran or other high-fibre cold cereals that have ten grams of fibre or more per serving. Though these cereals are not much fun in themselves, you can liven them up with fruit or fruit-flavoured fat- and sugar-free yoghurt or even sugar-reduced fruit spreads. If you wish to sweeten your cereal, use a sweetener, not sugar.

Cottage cheese

Low-fat or fat-free cottage cheese is an excellent high-protein food. Add fruit to it for a snack or add it to salads.

Eggs

During phase one you should limit your consumption of eggs to no more than half a dozen a week. These should preferably be omega-3 whole eggs because of their heart health benefits. However, you may use as many egg whites as you wish. In phase two you may eat within reason as many eggs as you like unless you have a medical cholesterol problem.

Fish/Shellfish

These are ideal green-light foods, low in fat and cholesterol and a good source of protein. Some coldwater fish such as salmon are also rich in omega-3. Never eat battered or breaded fish.

Food bars

Most food or nutrition bars are dietary disasters, high in carbohydrates and calories but low in protein. These bars are simply quick sugar fixes. There are a few, such as Myoplex or Protein Power Bars, that have a more equitable distribution of carbohydrates, proteins and fats. Look for 20 to 30 grams of carbohydrates, 12 to 15 grams of protein and 5 grams of fat. This comes to about 220 calories per bar. Keep them at home and at work for a convenient snack – remember that the serving size is half of one bar. In an emergency, it's okay to have one bar plus an apple and a glass of skimmed milk for lunch if you can't get away for a proper break. But try not to make a habit of it.

Grapefruit

One of the top-rated green-light foods. Eat grapefruit as often as you like.

Hamburgers

These are acceptable only if they have been made with extra-lean minced beef that has 10 per cent or less fat. You can add some oat bran to the meat to provide more fibre and less fat. Alternatively, you could use minced turkey or chicken. And there are some soy substitutes for meat that taste remarkably good and are worth checking out. Keep the serving size at 120g (4oz) and eat open-faced with only half of a wholemeal bun.

Meat

The best green-light meats are skinless chicken and turkey, fully trimmed beef, veal, deli cuts of lean ham, and back bacon. The beef cuts to choose are round, sirloin or tenderloin.

Milk

Use skimmed only. If you have trouble adjusting to it, then use semi-skimmed and slowly wean yourself off it. The fat you're giving up is saturated. Milk is a terrific snack or meal supplement. I drink two glasses of skimmed milk a day, at breakfast and lunch.

Nuts

Nuts are a principal source of 'good' fat, which is essential for your health. Almonds are your best choice. Add them to cereals, salads and desserts. Because they are calorie dense, they must be used in moderation.

Oat bran

You can use this excellent high-fibre food in baking as a partial replacement for flour, or you can make it into a hot cereal.

Oranges

Fresh oranges are excellent as snacks, at breakfast and added to cereals. A glass of orange juice has 2½ times as many calories as a whole orange, so avoid the juice and stick with the real thing.

Pasta

Most pastas are acceptable if you do not overcook them (pasta should be al dente, with some firmness to the bite) and if you limit the serving size to a quarter of your plate. Never use pasta as the basis of a meal – it is a side dish only.

Peaches, pears and plums

These fruits are terrific snacks, desserts or additions to breakfast cereal. Buy them fresh, or tinned in water or juice (drain the juice).

Porridge

If you haven't had porridge since you were a kid, now's the time to revisit it. Large-flake, or old-fashioned, porridge is the breakfast of choice, because not only is it green-light, but it also lowers cholesterol. The instant and quick cooking (one-minute) versions are not recommended because they have a far higher G.I. content due to the extra processing of the oats. I like porridge so much, I often have it as a snack with unsweetened apple sauce and sweetener (I use 30g [1oz] oats).

Potatoes

Only boiled new potatoes are acceptable on the G.I. Diet. They have a low starch content, unlike the larger, more mature potatoes, which are very red-light. Still, limit your quantity to two or three per serving.

Rice

Various types of rice have different G.I. ratings, and most of them are red-light. The best kinds are basmati and long grain, and brown is better than white. Don't overcook rice so that it starts to clump together. The more it's cooked, the more glutinous and red-light it becomes.

Soups

Tinned soups have a higher G.I. rating than homemade ones because of the high temperature at which commercial varieties are processed. I have included some brands of tinned soup in the green-light category because these are the best alternative available. Homemade soups are even more green-light.

Sour cream

Low-fat or fat-free sour cream with a little sweetener stirred in is an ideal alternative to whipped cream as a dessert topping. You can also mix fruit or low-sugar fruit spread into it for a creamy dessert.

Soy

Soy protein powder is a simple way to boost the protein level of any meal. It's particularly useful at breakfast for sprinkling over cereal. Look for the kind that has a 90 per cent protein content. It's sometimes labelled 'isolated soy protein powder'. Unflavoured low- or fat-free soya milk is a perfect green-light beverage.

Sweeteners (Sugar Substitutes)

There has been a tremendous amount of misinformation circulating about artificial sweeteners – all of which has been proven groundless. The sugar industry rightly saw these new products as a threat and has done its best to bad-mouth them. You can find an excellent medical overview of sweeteners in the U.S. Food and Drug Administration Consumer Magazine at www.fda.gov. Use, for example, Splenda or Hermesetas Gold to replace sugar in your diet. If you are allergic to sweeteners, then fructose is a better alternative to sugar. The herbal sweetener stevia, which can be found in health food stores, is acceptable if used in moderation since no long-term studies on its usage are available.

Tofu

Though not flavourful in itself, tofu can be spiced up in a variety of ways and is an excellent low-fat source of protein. Use it to boost or replace meat and seafood in stir-fries, burgers and salads.

Yoghurt

Non-fat, fruit-flavoured yoghurt sweetened with aspartame is a great green-light product and has one of the lowest G.I.s of all foods. It makes an ideal snack or a flavourful addition to breakfast cereal or fruit for dessert. I always keep our refrigerator well stocked with a variety of flavours. In fact, my shopping cart is so full of yoghurt containers that fellow shoppers frequently stop me to ask if they are on special!

Yoghurt cheese

A wonderful substitute for sour cream in desserts or in main dishes like chili. Emily has provided a recipe for this green-light staple on page 114.

Note: Additional updates can be found at **www.gidiet.co.uk.**

Appendix II
Green-Light Larder Guide

LARDER

BAKING/COOKING
Baking powder/soda
Cocoa
Dried apricots
Sliced almonds
Wheat bran
Wholemeal flour

BEANS (TINNED)
Baked (low-fat)
Mixed salad beans
Soyabeans
Vegetarian chili

BREADS
100% stone-ground wholemeal

CEREALS
All-Bran
Bran Buds
Fibre First
Porridge oats (large flake)

DRINKS
Bottled water
Club soda
Decaffeinated coffee/tea
Diet soft drinks

FATS/OILS
Rapeseed oil
Margarine (no-fat, light)
Mayonnaise (no-fat)
Olive oil
Salad dressings (no-fat)
Vegetable oil sprays

FRUIT (TINNED/BOTTLED)
Apple sauce (no sugar)
Mandarin oranges
Peaches in juice or water
Pears in juice or water

PASTA
Fettuccine
Spaghetti
Vermicelli
Penne

PASTA SAUCES
(VEGETABLE BASED ONLY)
Light sauces with no added sugar

RICE
Basmati
Long-grain
Wild

SEASONINGS
Flavoured vinegars/sauces
Spices/herbs

SNACKS
Food bars

SOUPS
(VEGETABLE OR BEAN-BASED ONLY)
Baxter's Healthy choice

SWEETENERS
Hermesetas Gold
Splenda

FRIDGE

DAIRY
Buttermilk
Cottage cheese (1%)
Fruit yoghurt (fat- and sugar-free)
Milk (skimmed)
Sour cream (fat-free or low-fat)

FRUIT
Apples
Blueberries
Blackberries
Cherries
Grapefruit
Grapes
Lemons
Limes
Oranges
Peaches
Pears
Plums
Raspberries
Strawberries

MEAT/POULTRY/FISH/EGGS
All seafood (no batter or breading)
Chicken breast (skinless)
Ham/turkey/chicken(lean deli)
Low-cholesterol omega-3 eggs
Turkey breast (skinless)
Veal

VEGETABLES
Asparagus
Aubergine
Beans (green or runner)
Broccoli
Peppers
Cabbage
Carrots
Cauliflower
Celery
Courgettes
Cucumber
Lettuce
Mangetout
Mushrooms
Olives
Onion
Peppers
Peppers (chilis)
Pickles
Potatoes (new only)
Radishes
Sugar snap peas
Spinach
Tomatoes

FREEZER

DAIRY
Ice cream (low fat and no added sugar)

SNACKS
Homemade muffins
(see recipes pp. 167–169)

VEGETABLES/FRUIT
Mixed berries
Mixed Fruit
Mixed peppers
Mixed vegetables
Peas

MEAT/POULTRY/FISH/EGGS
(See Fridge)

Appendix III
G.i. Diet Shopping List

LARDER

BAKING/COOKING
Baking powder/soda
Cocoa
Dried apricots
Sliced almonds
Wheat/oat bran
Wholemeal flour

BEANS (TINNED)
Baked beans (low-fat)
Mixed salad beans
Most varieties
Vegetarian chili

BREAD
100% stone-ground wholemeal

CEREALS
Bran Buds
Fibre First
Porridge oats (traditional large flake)
Soya protein powder

DRINKS
Bottled water
Club soda
Coffee/tea
Diet soft drinks

FATS/OILS
Almonds
Rapeseed oil
Margarine (no-fat/light)
Mayonnaise (no-fat)
Olive oil
Salad dressings (no-fat)
Vegetable oil spray

FRUIT (TINNED/BOTTLED)
Apple sauce (no sugar)
Mandarin oranges
Peaches in juice or water
Pears in juice or water

PASTA
Capellini
Fettuccine
Macaroni
Penne
Spaghetti
Vermicelli

PASTA SAUCES
(vegetable-based only)
Light with no added sugar

RICE
Basmati/long grain/wild

SEASONINGS
Flavoured vinegars/sauces
Spices/herbs

SNACKS
Food bars

FRIDGE/FREEZER

DAIRY
Buttermilk
Cottage cheese (low-fat or fat-free))
Ice cream (low-fat, no added sugar)
Milk (skimmed)
Sour cream (fat-free or low-fat)
Yoghurt (fat- and sugar-free)

FRUIT
Apples
Blackberries
Blueberries
Cherries
Grapefruit
Grapes
Lemons
Limes
Oranges
Peaches
Pears
Plums
Raspberries
Strawberries

MEAT/POULTRY/FISH/EGGS
All seafood (no batter or breading)
Chicken breast (skinless)
Extra lean ground beef
Ham/turkey/chicken (lean deli)
Liquid eggs (Break Free/Omega Pro)
Turkey breast (skinless)
Veal

VEGETABLES
Asparagus
Aubergine
Beans (green/runner)
Broccoli
Cabbage
Carrots
Cauliflower
Celery
Courgettes
Cucumber
Leeks
Lettuce
Mangetout
Mushrooms
Olives
Onions
Peppers (including chili)
Pickles
Potatoes (new/small only)
Sugar snap peas
Spinach
Tomatoes

SOUPS
Baxter's Healthy Choice

SWEETENERS
Hermesetas Gold, Splenda (and other sweeteners)

Appendix IV
G.i. Diet Dining Out Tips

BREAKFAST GREEN LIGHT
All-Bran
Egg Whites – Omelette
Egg Whites – Scrambled
Fruit
Porridge oats
Yoghurt (low-fat)

BREAKFAST RED LIGHT
Cold cereals
Bacon/sausage
Eggs
Scones
Pancakes/waffles

LUNCH GREEN LIGHT
Meats – deli style ham/
chicken/turkey breast
Pasta – ¼ plate maximum
Salads – low-fat
(dressing on the side)
Sandwiches – open-faced/
whole wheat
Soups – chunky vegetable-bean
Vegetables
Wraps – ½ wholemeal pita,
no mayonnaise

LUNCH RED LIGHT
Bakery products
Butter/mayonnaise
Cheese
Fast food
Pasta-based meals
Pizza/bread/bagels
Potatoes (replace with double
vegetables)

DINNER GREEN LIGHT
Chicken/turkey (no skin)
Fruit
Pasta – ¼ plate
Rice (basmati, brown,
wild, long grain) – ¼ plate
Salads – low-fat
(dressing on the side)
Seafood – not breaded or battered
Soups – chunky vegetable and bean
Vegetables

DINNER RED LIGHT
Beef/lamb/pork
Bread
Butter/mayonnaise
Caesar salad
Potatoes (replace with
double vegetables)
Puddings
Soups – cream based

SNACKS GREEN LIGHT
Almonds
Food bar – ½
Fresh fruit
Hazelnuts
Yoghurt – no fat/no sugar

SNACKS RED LIGHT
Chips, all types
Biscuits/Cakes/Scones
Popcorn, regular

PORTIONS
Meat – Palm of hand / Pack of cards
Rice/pasta – Maximum ¼ plate
Vegetables – Minimum ½ plate

Appendix V
The Ten Golden G.I. Diet Rules

1. Eat three meals and three snacks every day. Don't skip meals – particularly breakfast.

2. Stick with green-light products only in Phase I.

3. When it comes to food, quantity is as important as quality. Shrink your usual portions, particularly of meat, pasta and rice.

4. Always ensure that each meal contains the appropriate measure of carbohydrates, protein and fat.

5. Eat at least three times more vegetables and fruit than usual.

6. Drink plenty of fluids, preferably water.

7. Exercise for thirty minutes once a day or fifteen minutes twice a day. Get off the bus three stops early.

8. Find a friend to join you for mutual support.

9. Set realistic goals. Try to lose an average of a pound a week and record your progress to reinforce your sense of achievement.

10. Don't view this as a diet. It's the basis of how you will eat for the rest of your life.

G.I. DIET WEEKLY WEIGHT/WAIST LOG

WEEK	DATE	WEIGHT	WAIST	COMMENTS
1				
2				
3				
4				
5				
6				
7				
8				
9				
10				
11				
12				
13				
14				
15				
16				
17				
18				
19				
20				

Index